MW00790019

I was both informed and inspired, reading this book. Incorporate the wisdom and sage advice that is embedded in these pages and I am confident you will lead a more purposeful and fulfilling life. One whose foundation is of optimal health: physically, spiritually and beyond.

Sanjiv Chopra, MD, MACP, FRCP,
Bestselling Author
Professor of Medicine,
Harvard Medical School

Glenn's presence and unique perspectives integrate medicine, science, art and spirit in a way that stimulates mindfulness and brings joy to the reader. His inspiration and insights have a far-reaching impact, beyond what simple words can convey.

Eric W. McFarland, MD, PhD
Professor of Chemical Engineering
University of California, Santa Barbara

Before working with Dr. Glenn Wollman on personal healthcare issues, I often wondered what it would be like to receive care from a highly qualified physician who understood the critical importance of treating the whole person -- body, mind, heart and spirit. After decades of searching, I finally found that doctor. Dr. Wollman not only provided professional medical expertise, he responded to the human needs of my healing, and he did so with love.

Barbara Fields, Executive Director
Association for Global New Thought

Glenn's exceedingly brilliant yet empathetic and insightful approach to medicine made him the ideal guide for patients dealing with the complexities and intricacies of illness. Glenn understood the choices and priorities of care, and when to let healing happen without intervention.

Cory Gusland, MD

Dr. Wollman brings us the knowledge, experience, wisdom and clarity necessary to navigate the complexity of disease, illness and recovery. He is a physician, a medical scientist and a pioneer in the task of defining and impacting the mind-body-spirit.

Glenn makes the complex simple, distilling science down to the practical elements of eating, sleeping, breathing, connecting and creating. Words of true healing from a true healer.

Eddie Erlandson, MD
Co-Author of Radical Changes Radical Results
Former Chief of Staff at St. Joseph Mercy Hospital
Founder of Life Lessons

Dr. Glenn Wollman is the physician everyone dreams of having in their life. He possesses a rare combination of tremendous knowledge, deep wisdom, heartfelt concern and the ability to communicate all these with clarity, patience and precision.

Barbara De Angelis, PhD
New York Times Bestselling author

A Medical Guide's Road Map

YOUR PATH
of BEST
EXISTENCE

GLENN D. WOLLMAN, MD, WITH TRACEY DAVIS

ISBN: 979-8-9855634-5-0 (paperback)
ISBN: 979-8-9855634-0-5 (ebook)
Library of Congress Control Number: 2022944871

DISCLAIMER: *The contents of this book are for informational purposes
only and not intended to diagnose, treat, cure, or prevent any condition or
disease, nor to serve as a substitute for consultation with a qualified health-
care provider. The author and publisher of this book do not dispense medical
advice or prescribe any of these techniques as a form of treatment for physical,
emotional, or medical problems without the advice of a physician, either
directly or indirectly. Every effort has been made to ensure that the content
provided in this book is accurate and helpful for our readers at the time of
publishing. However, this is not an exhaustive treatment of the subjects. If
the reader requires personal medical, health, or other assistance or advice, a
competent professional should be consulted. The author, editors, and publisher
specifically disclaim all responsibility for any liability, loss, or risk, personal
or otherwise, that is incurred as a consequence, directly, or indirectly, of the
use and application of any of the contents of this publication.*

Printed in the United States of America.

Contents

PART THREE
Your Path: Navigating Health Care

PART FOUR
The Path of Questionable Existence:
A Dead End or a Cul-de-Sac?

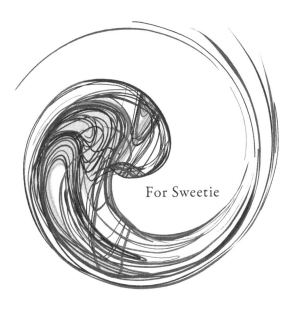

For Sweetie

By doing what you love, you inspire and awaken the hearts of others.

—*author unknown*

Introduction

I've held a beating heart in my hand.

How many people have been able to say that? Only a special group has had that unique privilege, yet I don't claim it boastfully. I say it humbly. Respectfully. Reverentially.

Physically, holding a human heart feels miraculous. But from an emotional and spiritual point of view, it was an overwhelming experience. The human heart is the stuff of poetry, music, and art—not to mention, it is the universal representation of love.

And I have held one in my hand.

How could that not reshape my perspective as I walk the path of my life?

We are all travelers on this planet. Even the planet is a traveler! Family, environment, government, culture, religion, and philosophy may influence our path, but the decisions and choices we make create either a travel adventure or a nightmare. Consider this book your travel guide—helping you make more informed decisions along the way.

In the field of medicine, science requires we set critical "standards of care." These provide roots and boundaries to the art of practicing medicine, and also give the patient confidence and reason to trust us. Assuming there is also a science and an art to life, it seems reasonable we should set personal "standards of care" for ourselves.

As we embark on our life's path, each of us is born with treasured goals I call a Gift, a Mission, and a Responsibility.

We are given the Gift of mind and consciousness—accompanied by a supporting cast of physical systems providing sensory input, movement, immunity, circulation, reproduction, digestion, excretion, and... the list is long. We are challenged to honor, appreciate, and understand the gift.

We are each either in a state of health or in a state of health care.

It is, therefore, a good idea to prepare and plan for how to exist in the best manner in each state.

So, bear with me, fellow travelers; I'll try to make this quick. But before we set out, it's important that you understand the lay of the land and a little bit about my background and why I've come to write this book.

After earning my medical degree in 1972, I spent most of my medical career in emergency medicine, cocreating the emergency department as you know it today. I also served as the medical director of a number of hospital-based emergency departments as well as a regional medical director for a national group.

While doing all this, I was drawn to what was then called complementary and alternative medicine, and I eventually started one of the first hospital-based integrative medicine programs in the country in Santa Barbara, California.

But following a severe automobile accident that brought an unexpected abrupt ending to my career as an emergency department doctor, I forged a new path as a Medical Guide. During my deeply personal work with patients, I have been inspired to offer my years of experiential information on obtaining, maintaining, and regaining optimal health.

At the behest of my wife, Heidi, I now share those realizations with you. What follows a collection of the memories, stories, insights, and knowledge gathered over a lifetime of listening, examining, and treating the maladies people endure—and observing the outcomes. This, of course, includes my own injuries, ailments, and disorders.

My hope is to offer some guideposts so that you can create your own individual path through life that is smooth, exciting, healthy, and successful.

Along with our Gift, we have a Mission to fulfill our destiny—essentially our life's purpose. A very important factor to consider is that you fulfill your Mission and not one that others want for you—or, in reality, for themselves. Becoming aware of your Mission as early as possible—bringing it into your daily consciousness—is a key aspect of a happy and fulfilled life. I was fortunate to realize my mission at a young age, and it made a great difference in my life. But getting it right is more important than getting it early.

By fulfilling our individual Mission, we serve not only ourselves but also humanity. Our society needs to attain a critical mass of happy people doing good. If you exude—and promote—happiness, you increase the "goodness quotient" of the world.

Finally, we have the Responsibility of maintaining optimal health and balance (physical, mental, and spiritual) in order to take advantage of our Gift and fulfill our Mission. This Responsibility is so important that if we don't handle it well, our bodies are very adept at sending us warning messages. It's when we ignore those messages that bad things happen.

There is no one perfect path that everyone must travel; we each achieve our best existence by traveling different paths. I discovered the experiences I'll share with you along my path, my Mission—my Path to Health. It's certainly the path I love and know best, but I also believe it is the most critical aspect of our journey that everyone needs to understand.

This information shouldn't be confined to only young adults or the older baby boomers. It should be for everyone interested in being healthy and having a good life. Much like

Star Trek's Captain Kirk in the Kobayashi Maru scenario—the no-win situation—I always believed that there were unseen options. Anyone interested in living a happy life with optimal health should learn this information as early as possible.

Most of us tend to put health on a back burner until we get ill or injured. Most of us need to get slammed in the face before we make healthy decisions. Think of the times you have had great plans for an evening or a vacation, and you suddenly became ill or injured. It doesn't have to be something catastrophic; a simple head cold can make you feel miserable enough to sit up and take notice of what your body is telling you.

This book endeavors to help you strive to embrace, fulfill, and balance your Gift, Mission, and Responsibility, so that you may travel Your Path of Best Existence.

Before we dive in, because I want you to get the most out of this book, let me explain how it's organized. The book is broken down into four main parts. The first part explores my background and gives you a little bit about who I am and how I became a Medical Guide. I share some of the twists and turns of my personal journey and my multiple experiences on both sides of the scalpel. My hope is that it provides you with several key takeaways: the context for what a Medical Guide is and how you may benefit from having someone knowledgeable about a wide variety of healing modalities on your team; a recognition of opportunities to make daily choices that will impact both your current and future health; and, perhaps most importantly, the knowledge that when faced with seemingly insurmountable odds at the time of a first diagnosis, or living with a debilitating condition for the rest of your life, you are not alone. There are others out there who can advocate for your wellness and help guide you along your path to recovery.

The second part of the book explores six aspects of health that we can all benefit from to ensure a happy, healthy future.

In Part Three we explore the path we will most likely all encounter at some point in our lives, how we as individuals should choose to navigate our health and health care. And the fourth and final part covers the end of one's path and opens you up to consider how the choices we make today affect the road ahead as we all step closer to the final chapter of our lives.

So, if you are the type of person who wants to skip the background and cut to the chase (and miss out on many of my humorous stories), you can go straight to Part Two and begin forming healthy habits immediately. If you're facing an immediate health problem and looking for options to begin the next part of your journey and medical exploration, dive directly into Part Three. Of course, after reading these, if you want to circle back and find out how I came to be a Medical Guide, it may make even more sense. Where you begin is up to you.

Much like hiking on a trail through a forest, throughout this book you will find signposts along the way that lead you to bonus sections that are accessible exclusively through my website, **GlennWollman.com** These are available to you as a reader and are designed to go hand-in-hand with this book.

So, there you have it. The choice is yours: start at the beginning or the middle, whichever you prefer. Whatever you decide, the important thing is to start today.

"I wish I'd known then what I know now" is a common statement by people lamenting decisions made at a time when all the facts weren't known. It implies that more information and better thinking skills would have made for better choices and better outcomes. Part of my motivation for writing this book is to present thoughts, ideas, and possibilities to consider. My hope is that the phrase "I wish I'd known then what I know now" goes through a metamorphosis to become "I'm glad I knew then... because I am really enjoying now!"

So, in this book, I'll guide you along the path of optimal health. When this path balances and intertwines with the choice of your Mission (career), both should actualize happiness and a life worth living. Along the way, we will make some pit stops, take some side roads, and enjoy a few vistas.

Let's begin our journey together. Keep reading, fellow wayfarers.

This is a wonderful day.
I've never seen this one before.

—*Maya Angelou*

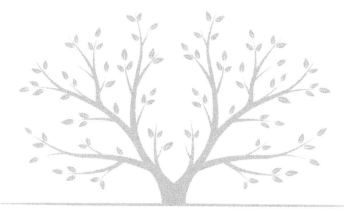

If you've forgotten the language of gratitude,
you'll never be on speaking terms with happiness.
—*author unknown*

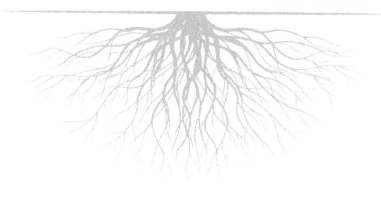

PART ONE

My Path:
Forging the Path of
Least Existence

If the path before you is clear,
you're probably on someone else's.

—*Professor Joseph Campbell, 1904–1987*

While I suggest the concept of taking a path that doesn't exist in order to move along your own path, it is important to have a good understanding of the paths that do exist. William Shakespeare had to learn the alphabet; Claude Monet had to learn about composition and color; martial artists have to learn horse stances and basic foundations. Once the basics were instilled, providing a solid foundation through intellect, each of these was able to move into their own consciousness allowing for the creative genius to emerge.

We may not all receive a Pulitzer Prize or have a painting in the Louvre, but we may achieve a state of balance and happiness that doesn't always come when one follows the existing paths, especially if it was not in our Mission and destiny.

This part will take you along the path I have taken.

Chapter One

"Carma"

For you numerologists, it was 03/30/03. I was leaving a dear friend's birthday party. As I got into my convertible and put the top down for a ten-minute ride on the 101 freeway, I began reflecting on how superb my life was. I had great friends, lived in a picturesque location, loved my home, and was fulfilling my dream job. I was deeply grateful for everything. Life couldn't get better.

My blood alcohol concentration level was zero; however, my blood apple juice level was slightly elevated (I'd had three glasses of juice). The beautiful night did not give any indication of how my life was about to change within the next few minutes.

I was hit by karma in the form of a car accident. My career in emergency medicine and my social and professional identities were obliterated in a "Santa Barbara second."

Preparing to exit the freeway, I heard a sickening crash. Within a nanosecond, I felt the hard impact at the back of my car. My car yawed to the left, shifting me into traffic—and I wasn't in control.

Time slowed—or at least my perception of it did.

To avoid traffic, I instinctively compensated by turning the wheel to the right. I missed the exit but hit a concrete marker—and went airborne. In my direct vision was a signpost and a tree directly behind it. (At the time, the tree looked like a forest.) I remember turning the steering wheel hard to the left—while in the air—futilely trying to avoid the oncoming obstacles.

I said to myself, "I may die now."

As my car slammed to the ground, I felt a severe pain in my lower back. The car immediately started sliding perpendicularly back across the freeway. A very strange cloudy, yellowish-gray light surrounded me. In the moment, it felt like a surreal, protective essence. (I later learned it was airbag residue.) Cars screeched past me both in front and behind—with horns blaring and brakes squealing.

Again I repeated, "I may die now."

The front of my car accordioned into the center divider, leaving the rear blocking the passing lane. As a good emergency physician, I checked myself over as well as I could. Everything hurt, especially my face, chest, and lower back. But I could move everything and was never unconscious.

Because mine was a dark-colored car, I knew other drivers hurtling toward me would have great difficulty seeing it. The car doors were jammed, so I couldn't get out. I was trapped.

Once more I said to myself, "I may die now."

It wasn't over. I heard the loud blasting horn of an eighteen-wheeler barreling toward me, brakes screaming. I wanted to move as far out of the way as possible, but because of the searing pain in my lower back, I could move my upper body only about two inches to the right. Now I was safe, right?

I laughed at the absurdity of it all.

The truck barely missed me, by such a slim margin I could feel my car being moved by the air pressure resulting from the truck's speed and bulk.

Eventually, two couples—Great Samaritans, by my estimation—stopped to help me. The door was bent, preventing them from opening it. I instructed them to lift me out. (I was so happy the top had been down.) They were hesitant, worrying about causing additional injuries, and queried, "Are you sure?"

I quickly told them, "We have no choice. We are all sitting ducks right now."

I didn't realize it at that moment, but it would soon become apparent that the life I had lived and loved for over thirty years—and the identity that I had developed over a lifetime—had all ended.

Paramedics showed up at the scene. Because I worked in the community, I knew them, and they all knew me. We had mutual respect for each other. I allowed them to check me over to confirm my assessment.

They offered to take me to the ED for a further workup. This may surprise you, but I declined. Why, you ask, would I make such a stupid decision?

Thank you for asking.

First, one of the most important and precious commodities in the emergency department was the beds—beds that needed to remain available for critical cases. I did not believe I had a surgical injury, and frankly, I didn't want to take up a bed. I also knew, because of my own body awareness and medical knowledge, I would seek help if my status changed.

Next, I knew they would be required to put me on a backboard and apply a protective cervical collar (a stabilizing neck brace to prevent a spinal cord injury). I knew that wasn't necessary from my own assessment, which the paramedics confirmed.

Third, I knew they would give me a lot of heavy-duty pain meds, such as morphine. That certainly would have helped my pain but would have interfered with a different type of healing that I believed was a priority.

For the record, I do NOT recommend refusing to go with the paramedics unless you feel completely capable of making the correct diagnoses based on medical training, internship, residency, and many years of practicing emergency medicine.

Eventually, I went to my emergency department and ordered lab tests to evaluate my persistent back pain. All of my tests were normal, except for the discovery of blood in my urine.

Aha! I probably had a kidney contusion, which answered the back pain and abnormally dark urine. After consulting with a radiologist, I decided to get a CT scan of my abdomen and back.

Diagnoses made:

Superficial facial lacerations, superficial chest and abdominal wall contusions, an ankle fracture, and burst compression fractures of my first and third lumbar vertebrae (from the impact of the crash landing).

I didn't expect the fractures, but the real shocker was that I was also passing my first kidney stone. I guess the Universe decided I wasn't in quite enough pain from my broken back.

I saw a neurosurgeon the next day who confirmed my assessment that I did not need surgery. However, I did need a body brace (which I wore for an extended period of time) in order for my two fractured lumbar vertebrae to heal properly.

While I was recovering from these multiple injuries, a dear friend was able to obtain some Chinese medicinal teas directly from Hong Kong. These contained scorpion parts as well as various healing herbs and were the sort of teas used by the Chinese army on the battlefield to prevent bleeding and accelerate wound healing.

Unfortunately, no matter how well I healed, my injuries were permanently limiting. My career in emergency medicine was over.

What was next?

None of the normal, traditional paths seemed exciting. I would either have to work in an urgent care or a clinical setting or start over in a different residency (perhaps psychiatry, so I wouldn't have to stand too much).

My thoughts came rapid-fire. Loved medicine; hated the idea of not being in the emergency department. Loved caring for people; hated the thought of working nine-to-five in a clinic. Loved treating gunshot wounds and stabbings; treating diaper rash just wouldn't cut it.

No practice or specialty in medicine existed that could accommodate my new physical issues and fill the all-encompassing chasm left by my traumatic departure from the ED.

Somewhat sad, mildly helpless, and admittedly a little scared, I went into a quiet space and meditated on my future.

What piece was missing from the medical jigsaw puzzle? What was lacking in medicine? How could I do my part to help heal, improve, and upgrade medicine?

These realities appeared in my meditations:

- Medicine is very complex and getting progressively more specialized, making it more difficult for any singular specialist to connect the dots.

- Doctors and patients don't always communicate effectively.

- Integrative and holistic practitioners and allopathic physicians rarely collaborate, if at all.

I realized that my skill sets were listening to people, making diagnoses, and either treating or triaging to other specialists.

Because of my extensive experience with both, I understood medicine as a doctor and a patient, therefore I could speak the languages of both. My knowledge of other cultural healing systems allowed me also to speak the languages of various holistic healers. I could be the bridge: interpreting, guiding, coordinating, and combining treatments. I could practice combinatorial medicine for optimal healing and health.

That was it! I would blaze a new trail and create a specialty that needed to exist, that of a Medical Guide. That was the missing piece of the jigsaw puzzle; instantly, the picture materialized.

I was on my newest path.

 For deeper insights into the trauma of this experience, visit **GlennWollman.com/resources** and check out Guidepost 15—Watch the Road Signs: Detour.

Chapter Two

The Silver Book

Although I have no true recollection, my parents—decidedly prejudiced and very proud of me—told me that I started walking at age six months. Clearly, I was already on my path.

My mother introduced me to love and humor. My father taught me discipline, how to live with pain, and magic, as he was an amateur magician. He also impressed upon me the importance of an education. Along with most of my family, he was an educator. He progressed from a physical education teacher to a fifth-grade elementary school teacher, to a school principal, to become involved on the county level as an administrator. Even after he retired, he worked tirelessly to develop a free, county-wide school transportation program for any child who didn't have a way of getting to school.

I remember going into my parents' bedroom, where my father had his library filled with all his books on education and some classic literature. They were all the usual colors of brown, umber, black, or deep red—mainly very dark, basically a blur—except for one, a lone book that was always on the highest shelf. I noticed it because it was silver in color, and it fascinated me. It was a supernova in a universe of darkness. I had no interest in any other book on the shelves.

When I was around six years old, he finally took it down from the shelf one day and showed it to me. It was a book on human anatomy from 1939, *Anatomical Studies for Physicians and Surgeons*, by Tom Jones. (No, not the singer.) I still remember my fascination and awe—even though I didn't know what the words *fascination* and *awe* meant—as I stared at the human skeleton and all the internal organs in glorious colors.

Until the age of nine, I don't remember having many thoughts on anything relevant. I was a kid: existing just for the day and whatever it brought.

There were no deaths in my family, not even a pet's, so I really had no understanding of life or death.

I was just eighteen months old when my brother was born. I didn't know when he arrived, where he came from, or his purpose. Eventually, over a decade later, I had a sister and a second brother. When they appeared, I understood a bit more, but I pondered nothing philosophical.

I had no idea there were important thoughts inside of me until seeing that silver book. It opened my consciousness; I began to realize things.

I never stopped thinking about it and constantly badgered my father to bring down the silver book for us to view. I don't know why, but my memory is that he took it down only once a year. But it seemed he took it down frequently, and each time he did, I was becoming more interested in anatomy, and my path was being forged.

I had made my decision to be a medical doctor. Of course, my parents were happy, but they actually tried to talk me out of it. At the time, doctors were still making house calls and were always being called for emergencies. My mother didn't want me to have that kind of life. She tried to steer me toward dentistry—a profession she considered less stressful. Little did she know that three-score-and-some fortnights later, dentists would have one of the highest rates of suicide in the health-care professions.

But in that decision-making moment, I eliminated a lifetime of anxiety and stress surrounding the proverbial adult questions: "What are you going to be when you grow up? Where are you going to college? What courses will you take? What will you major in?" The uncertainty was all gone, answered, gift-wrapped. Life was now a cool stroll, except, of course, for the fact that I would have to study a lot and be continually available to help others—for the rest of my life.

I didn't realize the enormous benefit at the time, but that knowledge of my future allowed me to start early on this path of least existence. What I mean is, I had the time to explore various philosophies, religions, and healing systems happening in other parts of the planet. I was drawn to the East and began appreciating its philosophies, martial arts, music, art, literature, and ancient practice of medicine.

In retrospect, a childhood obsession with that book on the highest shelf in my father's library became the trailhead for my life's path. Hmmm, maybe every kid should have their own version of a silver book.

Chapter Three

The Ceremony

Everyone has been made for some particular work, and the
desire for that work has been put in every heart.

—*Rumi*

It was 1958. Our family's good friend, Dr. Theodore Struhl, a general surgeon, knew that I was interested in a career in medicine. Hoping I might become a surgeon and one day take over his practice, he began my initiation when I was in junior high school.

It happened at midnight. I heard my parents' phone ring. Dr. Struhl informed them he was about to perform an emergency appendectomy and asked if I would like to observe.

I was so excited I could hardly breathe.

My father drove me to the hospital, where Dr. Struhl was waiting for me in the parking lot. As my father left, Dr. Struhl escorted me through the daunting doors of this great edifice. I followed him with uncontrolled anticipation as we made our way through the labyrinthian halls of the hospital, far into its depths. It was magical for me.

Entering the surgical dressing room, we both changed into our ceremonial gowns, surgical scrubs, hats, booties, and masks. We entered a room where we began a traditional cleansing ceremony, preparing ourselves for a very special ritual that was about to commence. Following very carefully and trying to mimic the technique of The Master, I used special soap—cleansing everything from my fingernails up past my elbows, making sure that everything became sterile. The process was lengthy; it seemed like an eternity. Each cleansed area could no longer touch anything else, or the entire scrub would have to be repeated.

Maybe I took a breath at this moment.

We quietly entered a mystical room. The air and the light were ethereal. It seemed almost futuristically cave-like, far away from the rest of the world. Although it was sterile, it held so many fascinating things to look at, but I kept my eyes slightly down because I didn't want to bring attention to myself: a twelve-year-old being allowed to witness this secret, special healing ceremony.

We were both approached by a group of attendants. Later on, I realized the incredible things that nurses do in every part of a hospital and in all of health care. They helped us into the ceremonial robes of the Medicine Shamans.

My head was already spinning when I finally realized a human body was lying on the special altar. The ritualistic ceremony to remove something evil from his body was about to commence. At age twelve, I was about to observe an emergency appendectomy on a young boy—a boy exactly my age. He would never know the impact he would have on the rest of my life.

Before going to the hospital, I had a few moments to read a little about the appendix in my parents' encyclopedia. This, by the way, was pretty much the source of all my knowledge and all book reports through high school. How great would it have been for my endlessly curious mind to have had computer and internet access at that time?

We approached the young body with the angry organ and began to do special incantations and cleansing ceremonies— preparing the body for a human entrance with a very sharp instrument. I didn't know what would happen when the incision was made. Would there be blood everywhere and might all the organs jump out at me?

I was about to see—for real—what had only been illustrated in a silver-colored book.

The next morning, tired but exhilarated, I was scheduled to give a talk to my class on something important in my life. Guess what I chose as my topic?

Years later, because of my original exposure to anatomy and the influence of our family friend, I eventually applied to medical school with plans to become a surgeon.

Chapter Four

The Thick Letter

If you're not excited about it, it's not the right path.

—anonymous

George H. Paff, PhD, was the legendary professor of anatomy and the head of the Admissions Committee at the University of Miami School of Medicine (now known as the Miller School of Medicine) in Miami, Florida. He was known for being tough, and I had an interview with him. All at once, I was completely excited and in utter terror. My entire life's dream, since age nine, had to pass through this one man.

He perused my application, records, grade-point average, MedCat entrance exam, and letters of recommendation, taking an excruciatingly long time. He finally looked up and asked, "Why should I let you become a doctor?"

Knowing I was preparing for a life as a surgeon and anticipating this question, I responded rapidly, "I love helping people, and I love working with my hands."

He responded with equal speed, "You should consider becoming an auto mechanic."

With those words, I felt as if I were in one of the old Samurai movies. You know the ones—where the voices don't match the lip movements. They all seem to share one similar scene:

The famous warrior wields his Katana blade, expertly targeting the neck of the evil warlord. After an effortless, almost motionless strike, the victim displays no movement and no expression for a seemingly infinite moment. Suddenly, a trickle of blood oozes around his neck. His expressionless head falls to the ground, and the rest of his body slumps.

Yep, that was how I felt. The sudden thought of becoming anything other than a doctor triggered the feeling that blood had begun oozing around my neck and my head was about to fall off.

The interview was over. Now I just had to wait for the thin letter of rejection or the thick letter of acceptance.

Obviously, I got the thick letter.

Chapter Five

Cadaver Chronicles

I have learned this at least by my experiment: that if one advances confidently in the direction of his dreams, and endeavors to live the life which he has imagined, he will meet with success unexpected in common hours.

—Henry David Thoreau

A varied, multicultural group of about a hundred students gathered in an ancient auditorium in a decrepit building.

We were the University of Miami School of Medicine's illustrious Class of 1972. (At least we thought we were illustrious... and still do!)

We were the last class to start our personal medical journeys in this building. The next year, all the medical students would move into a newly built, modern facility.

We all wore some version of the required uniform: white shirt, tie, white pants, and white shoes.

We all experienced the common knowledge of medical students: on day one, you are already six to eight weeks behind in your studies.

Each professor believes that their field is the most important one you need to know. They give out assignments for reading as if no other lecturers were going to give any at all. Imagine reading eight lengthy chapters, filled with multisyllabic words, usually long Latin or chemical names. Believe me, every word in my text was highlighted.

But I digress. Back to class.

Our very first class was anatomy, taught by a man you've already met, Dr. George Paff. (Remember the guy who thought I should be an auto mechanic?)

Aside from being a brilliant anatomist, he was incredibly important to our future. If you didn't pass his class, your chances of finishing medical school were slim. His style of teaching was demanding; he had no problem publicly berating those not prepared for the daily anatomy lecture. There were so many horror stories handed down by the upper classes that every medical student who took his class was in a state of abject terror even before we entered his classroom on day one.

Even as we were trying to absorb the most vital things we would ever learn, looming in the back of our minds—as well as in the adjoining room—were our cadavers. Most students learn their professions through lectures. Very few learn from cadavers.

We walked quietly into the cadaver lab, an old, un-air-conditioned room on a typical, muggy Miami day. Each of us was in somber silence as the blast of formaldehyde odor made us all wince and tear. As our eyes focused on the center of the room, we saw multiple metal tables. Along the sides of the room were the metal containers, each containing a corpse.

Opening the lid of each container compounded the burning smell with more formaldehyde. We divided ourselves into groups of four, were assigned a cadaver, transferred it from the locker, and placed it on our table. We felt a cyclone of emotions: fear, anticipation, fear, eagerness... and did I mention fear?

Before we started our dissections, Dr. Paff pointed out that each cadaver was a person. They had offered their bodies to us, ultimately saying, "Take me apart without fear or worry about putting me back together, so that you can learn how to put others back together."

Imagine for one moment how it might transform you to spend every day for several months with a formerly live human being, taking it apart tissue by tissue. It's a transformative experience.

What a blessing! I honor all those who chose to be cadavers by donating their bodies to science for the sake of humanity. The rest of my career utilized that special knowledge to help others begin their lives, live their lives, or end their lives.

A couple of asides from the Cadaver Chronicles:

- We all eventually got used to the formaldehyde.

- And my experience in the cadaver lab gave me an unintended gift: if, on occasion, while eating a meal with others, someone might begin a conversation with the disclaimer "This may not be a suitable topic while eating," I can confidently respond, "I ate many meals while working on my cadaver; nothing you can say will ruin my appetite!"

Chapter Six

Squid Ink

As I mentioned before, we were a varied group: approximately ninety-one men and nine women. We were mostly white with some Hispanics (primarily Cuban) and a few Middle Easterners. We were of varying degrees of intelligence; some were on a special track (on an MD PhD program). Most had aspirations toward future specialties, and some had no idea.

Some were married—with or without children—some single. Our ages ranged from early to midtwenties up through midforties. We held varied political beliefs, religions, and ideologies.

We rarely agreed on anything outside of medicine.

I was among the small group labeled "The Hippies." We had long hair and beards and loved rock and roll. Hippies, schmippies. Above anything else, we were first-year medical students and had work to do.

After a brief time, it was fairly easy to know who the "brains" in the class were and who were the "brown-nosers," always eager to ask a question to which they already knew the answer. Soon, one could hear the groans in the class when their hands went up. Even the professors recognized them.

Not everyone graduated. To its credit, once the medical school committed to a student, it tried very hard to keep them on track and in the program until completion. Despite this support, not everyone reached the finish line.

Some dropped out because of poor grades and difficulty keeping up with the intensity and massive amount of work.

Some dropped out because of the pressure and the realization that being a doctor was not really their Mission (probably someone else's dream for them that they were trying to fulfill).

Of those who graduated, many went into private practice. Some became highly respected and innovative in their fields at prestigious hospitals and medical centers. Some went into the military; some relocated to rural areas and made a difference for those communities; some dove into research. Some are still practicing; others have retired or died. One thing is for sure: there never was nor will there be a class like ours (purely unbiased observation, of course).

I see new doctors beginning their practices today, and they are practicing a different type of medicine. For our class and a few after us, it was about the relationship with our patients. We were trained to take a really good history and do a really thorough physical examination to come up with a differential or specific diagnosis. And we depended on ancillary departments, such as the lab and radiology, to either rule in or rule out our diagnoses.

Many of today's doctors—although in fairness, not all—are not as interested in the doctor-patient relationship, nor in a deep history and physical exam. Because the technology is much better now, the new breed is focused on diagnosis based on technology. They believe listening to the chest with a stethoscope is not always as accurate as a CT scan or MRI of the chest. While this may be correct, I believe leaving out the human touch eliminates an opportunity to promote the very precious bond between the doctor and their patient.

As a Medical Guide, I am careful to determine what type of doctor my clients prefer, as I help match them with a healer. "Would you prefer a doctor who will first use a stethoscope or order an MRI?" Their answer provides an important personal preference.

As I said before, our class rarely agreed on anything, but we did come together on two specific occasions. The first occurred in a laboratory biochemistry class. It was a class requiring understanding and memorization of an inordinate number of chemical names, equations, and formulas. Adding to the demands of the class, the textbook was written by our professor.

We were approaching a critical midterm exam, covering a great many chapters in the text. As it turned out, the professor departed from the usual testing procedure. He took absolutely none of the questions from the main reading material, and instead took all the questions from the footnotes (a somewhat inappropriate and definitely rude procedure). Almost everyone, including the A students and the brown-nosers, failed it. This was unheard of and unacceptable—especially to those obsessed with getting an A.

As a class, we went to the dean and presented our case. Lowly medical students versus a tenured, respected professor. The odds were against us. Our solution was to take a makeup test consisting of questions from the body of the book—not from the footnotes. Additionally, the professor had to provide a list of a hundred questions from which he would pick fifty for the test.

Our class came together. And, lo and behold, we prevailed!

I said there were two things that unified us. The other was surprisingly nonmedical: a popular television cooking show, *The Galloping Gourmet*, featuring Graham Kerr. We all spent many of our lunch hours in the TV room. Each of us counted on someone's willingness to stay until the end of the show—and take the hit for being late to class—to write down the recipe of the day for the rest of the class. I remember clearly, I supplied the recipe for Shrimp and Noodles with a Squid Ink Sauce.

Chapter Seven

From Cadavers to Totem Poles

In my third year of medical school, we still attended classroom lectures—trying to learn everything currently known about the inner workings of the species we would soon be treating in whatever specialty we chose. But now we would also rotate through all of the different major medical services, such as general and internal medicine, surgery, obstetrics, pediatrics, and so forth. For the first time, we were on the wards, meeting and taking care of real people—without any smell of formaldehyde.

But, since none of us really knew anything about actually taking care of living humans, we were the part of the medical totem pole that was buried underground. Older, more experienced medical students, followed by interns, residents, chief residents, attendings, fellows (an advanced degree of training), medical staff, heads of departments, the chief of staff, professors, and the dean of the medical school, were the totem pole in the big picture.

As a third-year medical student on a surgical rotation, I was called to the emergency room to see a patient.

At that time, the "room" was completely different from today's emergency department. Remember, this was a time when there was no specialty in emergency medicine. In those days, emergency rooms were merely a designated area within the hospital to attend to urgent needs. There were no distinct protocols. The rooms were predominantly staffed by moonlighting residents who were in school while trying to raise a family. (They needed the extra money!)

I walked in to see the patient, a frightened twelve-year-old boy with a palm frond stuck in his right eye. The part sticking out of his eye was at least two feet long, and we had no idea how far into his eye it had penetrated.

His family was scared out of their minds.

Of course, at this point in my training, I had absolutely no idea what to do except consider the totem pole. I immediately called the fourth-year medical student, who also had no idea what to do.

We called our intern. No idea.

We called all the first-, second-, and third-year residents. No ideas.

We finally called the chief resident, who at least had an idea. He thought about pulling it out directly, but decided to first check with the ophthalmologist.

The ophthalmologist said, "Don't touch it without first doing X-rays to see the extent of penetration." (Remember, CAT scans and MRIs didn't exist yet.)

From the X-rays, we determined that the errant frond went in about two or three inches into the eye socket, but, amazingly, seemed to miss the eye!

By now we were at least two hours after his admission. I felt all at once fascinated and helpless. The only thing I was qualified to do was offer support to the patient and his mother and provide encouragement that everything would be okay (and even that was something I was still in the process of learning during my initial training in "bedside manner").

After the X-rays, the ophthalmologist decided he didn't want to touch it and decided to call the neurosurgeon.

The neurosurgeon, after looking at the films and examining the child, felt optimistic the palm frond could be removed, but he didn't want to touch it either.

It was good for me to watch the wheels of medicine. Decisions and consults and gathering data were all in motion, but there was still a palm frond in the kid's eye.

After about three hours, the chief surgical resident walked in. He unceremoniously grabbed the palm frond, and as we all gasped in terror, he simply pulled it out. No fanfare, no nothing. No palm frond.

The boy was admitted, was watched for a few days, and went home without incident—just some scary memories and lasting lessons for a twelve-year-old child and a twenty-four-year-old medical student. (Little did I know, a seed had been planted that emergency medicine would be where I would bloom.)

At the top of the totem pole on the actual wards—where medicine was carried out—were the nurses. Possibly the most important thing I learned in medical school was to trust, respect, and listen to THE NURSES! (Although, just as an aside, they also had their own totem pole.)

While performing a surgical procedure, the attending surgeon would ask us questions about differential diagnosis, procedures, and anatomy (pointing to some tissue and demanding its name, blood supply, nerve supply, and function). This interrogation was obviously done in front of more advanced students, other surgeons, and nurses. Of course, the primary goal was our learning, but the secondary purpose was to force us to think and act under extreme physical and mental pressure. Consequently, the questions kept coming until we eventually arrived at a question to which we had to answer, "I don't know."

Sometimes at this point, the surgeon would look over at a nurse and ask her the same question. Of course, the nurse had likely assisted in these procedures for years and had watched all of us nervous, young students eventually get the wrong answer.

The nurse always had the correct answer. In many ways, the nurses taught us as much as the doctors (and still do).

I was excited during my three-month surgical rotation. This was my path. I was ready.

The schedule was easy to remember:

- Make rounds at 5:00 a.m. on all patients scheduled for surgery that day and draw blood work.

- Be ready for surgery at 7:00 a.m. Plan to assist, observe, accept being berated, and learn.

- Continue operating throughout the day—except when there are scheduled lectures.

- After surgery, make rounds on post-op patients, and then examine the new patients for tomorrow's surgeries.

When we were finished, usually in the late evening, we were free to go home, eat, study, and sleep—usually all at the same time—in order to be ready at 5:00 a.m. to start again.

Unless we were on call.

While on call, we slept at the hospital. (And I use the word *slept* quite loosely. We hardly ever slept because we were the first ones to be called when anyone higher on the totem pole needed something done during the night.) I was on call so often, there were long stretches in which I would lose all awareness of the outside world. Inevitably, a fellow student who had not been on call would shake me back into reality.

They might greet me with something like "How was your Fourth of July celebration?"

Only at that moment would I realize it was no longer June.

I didn't mind; I was in my element. I loved medicine so much, I could have talked about it every minute of every day—I'm still that way.

The problem was, as I rotated through each of the services—pediatrics, obstetrics and gynecology, internal medicine, and all the other subspecialties—I realized that I really loved all of them—not only the knowledge but also working with the people in each field. This caused an internal dilemma because no matter which specialty I chose, I would not be able to continue learning and treating people in all the different areas.

Chapter Eight

"Happy Birthday to You!"

When I was going through my obstetrics rotation, I was introduced to one of the experiences I would come to love and knew I would miss if I chose another specialty: childbirth.

Now, of course, I don't mean I had the experience of *having* a child. What I'm talking about is the act of *delivering* a child.

There is nothing like it from many aspects:

- Briefly getting to know the expectant mother and her views on preparing for the delivery and parenting

- Observing how each mother uniquely dealt with the process and the pain

- Getting to know the expectant family—Mom's partner as well as occasionally other siblings

- The entire delivery process: determining which part of the baby is going to come out first; feeling the head and internal pelvic landmarks to calculate the passage through the birth canal; working with the mother to promote passage while not causing harm by moving too quickly; protecting my two patients from damage caused by too much force at the wrong time

- It's mesmerizing when the head, the face, or another part begins to crown and present itself to the new world.

- Assessing the vital signs of the baby, its first breath, its steady heartbeat

- Cutting the vital cord—officially removing the child's tie to its mother, declaring independence and individuality

- Cleaning and warming the child

- Introducing mother and child to each other for their first visual contact and embrace

So many great memories.

Through many deliveries over the years, some simple and some complex, I realized one critical thing was missing: even though this is the *only* time it will happen and the *only* real time it is appropriate, no one ever sang "Happy Birthday"!

Later in my career in the emergency department, I started doing just that.

Chapter Nine

The "Mirror, Mirror on the Wall" Rotation

During my general surgery rotation, I had an opportunity to work on two plastic surgery cases. It just so happened that our hospital employed a world-renowned plastic surgeon and offered a world-class program. It was so world-class, in fact, that after one had finished four years of medical school and four years of general surgery, there was a *ten-year* waiting list to get into the program!

The first case that deeply influenced me involved a young adult who was simply walking on a Miami sidewalk when a high-power electrical wire broke, swung down, and hit him directly in the face. It literally *melted* his entire face.

Over many years and many surgeries, the plastic surgery department had been rebuilding his face (as an example, taking cartilage from a rib to create ears and a nose). From a medical point of view, it was fascinating. From every other point of view, it was... well, almost macabre.

The second influential case was much more direct. A middle-aged homeless man, sleeping on a railroad track, was momentarily awakened by the sound of his facial bones being split apart. From his front hairline to his chin—in a direct line between his eyes, through his nose and mouth—he was left with a three-quarter-inch gap down the middle of his face.

Not seeing myself operating on hernias and gallbladders for the rest of my life—and being an artistic type of guy—I found myself leaning toward this creative subspecialty as a potential new path. I signed up for an elective rotation on the plastic and reconstructive surgical service.

Surgery, Sex, and Stethoscopes

Each late afternoon, a group of us gathered at the central nurses' station on the postsurgical ward. We were the chief attending physician, the chief resident, the other residents, the fellows (a level of study, not a gender), and I (the only medical student and therefore, as you now know, lowest on the totem pole). Part of my assignment was to precede the team, remove surgical dressings and bandages from the patients, and prepare and present each patient to the rest of the team once they arrived.

My first patient was a beautiful woman recovering from a minor cosmetic procedure. As a twenty-five-year-old, fourth-year medical student, I wasn't trained to notice a glaring warning sign: she was reclining in the bed, wearing a sexy teddy—not a hospital gown.

After introducing myself, I proceeded to remove the surgical dressing from behind her ear. Before I knew it, she was gripping my stethoscope (which I wore draped casually around my neck) and was pulling me down so I was on top of her! In an instant she was kissing me.

That was the view the team of doctors saw when they entered the room on afternoon rounds.

I never wore my stethoscope that way again.

Chapter Ten

A Timely Kidnapping

It was a beautiful, sunny spring Miami afternoon, and I was returning from lunch, headed back toward the medical school auditorium for an afternoon lecture on epidemiology. A friend of mine came up from behind me, put her arm in mine, and said, "I'm kidnapping you and taking you to my favorite hotel on Miami Beach for lunch."

Boring lecture on epidemiology... lunch?

Lunch... epidemiology?

Oh, what to do?

Because I loved medicine so much, I was leaning toward the lecture, but her proposition and my mental fantasy were so strong that I found myself in her car going over the causeway to Collins Avenue.

Entering the lobby of the hotel, I started to get a little hungry and began looking forward to a great feast. It was at that moment that I saw a large sign announcing what appeared to be the first conference on emergency medicine. I didn't even know what that meant!

You see, at the time, emergency rooms were not staffed in the way we think of them today. They were covered by residents and starving interns who were trying to supplement their income to support a new family or pay off their student loans. There was no specialty that existed.

My interest became so completely piqued that my earlier plans for the afternoon waned from my consciousness.

As I walked into the hall, they immediately gave me a gift of a vinyl attaché case with the words *Emergency Medicine* embossed on it. Those words hit me like a bolt of lightning. And that's when I realized *this* was my new specialty—a path that didn't yet exist.

Chapter Eleven

The Path of Least Existence

Do not go where the path may lead, go instead where there is no path and leave a trail.

—*Ralph Waldo Emerson*

I changed my course from plastic and reconstructive surgery to emergency medicine.

Since this was a brand-new area of medicine—not yet a specialty—I had to design my own unique educational path. I constructed a surgical internship and residency to prepare myself for a career in emergency medicine.

Westward ho, Los Angeles, California!

I had no desire to become a surgeon anymore but knew that surgical knowledge and skills would be vital in the emergency department. Through this surgical internship and residency, I would learn how to diagnose an acute surgical condition, become proficient with all the instruments of a surgeon, and master suturing techniques that would help me—and benefit my patients—time and time again in the emergency department.

I also learned valuable lessons about dealing with emotional roller coasters and judgment.

Things Aren't Always As They Seem

One afternoon, in the second year of my surgical residency, I was making rounds with the other surgical interns, residents, and our attending. Unexpectedly, I was called to the emergency department for a trauma case. I was informed it was an auto versus pedestrian, and the pedestrian was an eleven-year-old boy.

I arrived in the ED at the same time as the ambulance. The child was in bad condition. He was unconscious and needed to be intubated, so I quickly placed a tube into his trachea.

Using an instrument in my left hand to control the mouth and tongue and expose the vocal cords, I held the tube with my right hand, ready to place it between the vocal cords and into the main windpipe. This is a critically important skill to learn—and *perfect*—if you are going to work in an emergency department.

A trained respiratory therapist assisted the patient's breathing, using a bag connected to the tube I had just inserted. The nurses started intravenous lines, collected blood for the lab, and placed a Foley catheter into the patient's bladder. His vital signs (blood pressure, pulse, and respirations) were in critical ranges. Not only did we need to move quickly to get him to surgery; he also needed blood.

The most obvious injuries were complete amputations of one arm and the opposite leg. Both remaining extremities were severely damaged, and we weren't sure if they could be saved. We evaluated for internal damage in the chest and abdomen and looked for injuries to the brain and spinal cord as we prepared the surgical team: both an orthopedic surgeon and a general surgeon.

It was heartbreaking for all of us to see this young child with such devastating injuries. We couldn't help but project what his future might be like—if he survived.

Before we took him to surgery, the police showed up and told us that the accident *was* no accident. It was purposeful. Someone had tried to run him over!

We were confused and couldn't justify something like that. Who would do this to a young kid, and why?

But the next piece of information we received blew us away. Our innocent victim was actually a member of a local gang—in fact, was a *hit man* for the gang. (Because minors could not be tried in court as adults, it was one of the policies of the gang to utilize young boys as murderers.)

This child–hit man, we were informed, had already been involved in multiple gang shootings, and a member of one of those rival gangs had been driving the vehicle that mowed him down.

Now we were angry. Now we had some understanding of the justification behind this attack. But even with all our emotions in a tailspin, as professionals, we let it all go and went about the task of saving an *individual*.

The surgery was complex and took many hours, but it appeared we were getting a handle on his condition and were going to save him. I guess we were hoping that this catastrophe would possibly help him—and even other members of his gang—change their ways, become better citizens, and stop the violence. (We were young and still idealistic.)

As we were closing, the chief surgeon asked me to go out to the waiting room and inform the family of his critical—but stable—status. (Communicating highly emotional and sometimes uncomfortable information was an indispensable part of my training.)

I met with his mother, who was obviously scared. Standing around her were some of his siblings and friends (or possibly fellow gang members). Everyone was nervous and wanted details.

I gave them the good news that he was going to be okay, and they would be able to see him later in the critical care unit. Relief and joy lit up the waiting room.

Mere moments later, one of the OR nurses came out, took me aside, and said, "The child had a cardiac arrest and died."

I had no way to anticipate the myriad of feelings I would experience as I helped create a brand-new specialty in an ancient profession. I had no idea of the things I would see over the years—the best and the worst of humanity.

I finished my augmented surgical internship and residency at a hospital in downtown Los Angeles. I thought I was totally ready for the ER. In reality, I had only a minimal appreciation of *how* to be an emergency room doctor, the rigors of an entire shift alone—as "The Doctor"—without any fellow residents or attendings to back me up and help me make the correct decisions.

You see, as I said before, when I decided on a career in emergency medicine, it wasn't a specialty at all. It was as the name *emergency room* implied—merely a room within the hospital, nothing like it is today. A very large, courageous (albeit strange) group of doctors and nurses were drawn to that field. We worked very hard to gain specialty status within the entire medical field.

Being a "room," we weren't recognized by the specialists. Hospital staff meetings didn't include representatives from "rooms"—only departments. Only departments were on the Medical Executive Committee that made policy decisions.

We pushed to join! We were confident we belonged because all the represented departments were related to us. We interacted with every one of them. We needed an equal voice.

They saw us as marauding hordes invading their department privilege. Existing doctors tried to fight us, saying in essence, "You don't need to be a department. Just go to your room." But we needed to have our own writings, data, and language.

Being eventually recognized as a department by the American Medical Association was a big deal.

As a burgeoning specialty, we took on the "crisis" elements of every other specialty. We became experts in making life-and-death decisions—rapidly and repeatedly. As a group we also began to question many of the widely accepted, long-standing treatments. In doing so, we were able to improve treatments in many of the other specialties.

We left our "room" and created the "emergency department."

I'm very proud of what we accomplished.

Bennies

I spent over thirty years in the emergency department (affectionately called "The Pit" by those of us in this new field).

Over the course of my career, I worked in small, rural EDs, exclusive Beverly Hills hospitals, and major trauma centers.

If I were to write down all the perks of practicing emergency medicine, the list would probably stretch from Santa Barbara to Miami. But for the purpose of our conversation here, I'll condense the list to the major benefits I received.

Emergency medicine

- gave me the opportunity to learn the stories of people's lives and their experiences;

- taught me how to ask important questions without fear;

- taught me how to listen;

- allowed me to confidently approach painful topics;

- instilled in me the value of appreciating moments;

- made me recognize the fragility—and narrow margins—between health and illness, and between life and death;

- taught me how to wash my hands so they are really clean!

- empowered me to feel comfortable during an emergency or at the scene of an accident; and

- gave me the skill to repair a few things that require sewing, although I have to suture with instruments.

From an economic, social, and public health point of view, I had the great pleasure to order whatever I thought necessary on behalf of my patient, without prior approval, third-party requirements, complicated forms, or distant appointments potentially at another facility. I didn't appreciate this benefit much at the time, but in light of the various worldviews of health care that have followed my years of practice, it indeed was a blessing!

I was able to procure the tests and specialist interpretations, and have almost instantaneous consults at the patient's bedside. This nimble reaction time allowed rapid decision-making and equally rapid application of my healing strategy.

Emergency was really a special opportunity to practice medicine in its best form.

Don't Judge before Taking the History

Many people ask the question "How's life treating you?"

From the point of view of taking a good history, that seems to be an excellent question to find out pertinent information quickly.

But perhaps even more enlightenment can come from one follow-up question: "How are you treating life?"

In the ED, life-and-death decisions rely on a quick—and, most importantly, accurate—diagnosis. This, of course, cannot be achieved without taking a thorough history.

One of the real-life benefits of practicing emergency medicine is realizing it's the same thing with other sorts of judgments: you need to take a good history before making one!

As the medical director of the emergency department, I received complaints from patients, families of patients, nurses, other hospital staff, and basically anyone who found me. It was part of the job.

One morning as I came in for a day shift, I was approached by a fairly irate doctor. "Your nursing staff screwed up last night with one of my private patients!" he bellowed.

I remained silent and listened intently—an excellent strategy to field complaints.

"Your department referred my patient to another doctor last night for follow-up. This can't happen again! You need to do something about your nurses!" (Actually not officially "my" nurses.)

"Please give me the name of the patient, and I will find out what happened. I'll get back to you with a plan to make provisions and policy so that this type of event does not occur again," I said sincerely.

I began my research, looking up the incident, checking the patient's medical record, speaking with the ED doctor who treated the patient, speaking with the nurses and the staff of clerks, and finally speaking with the patient on record.

I had my answer to the problem.

I called the still-irate doctor. "I hope you found out who screwed up!" he emphatically stated.

"I did. After doing much research and speaking with everyone, I learned that this is what happened: Your patient asked for you to be called. Our staff called. You didn't answer. We called your answering service. They were also unable to get in touch with you. Your answering service told us that you had turned off your beeper and could not be reached. After multiple attempts, the furious patient requested a new doctor."

A long silence ensued on the other end.

Then, finally, I heard a quiet "Oh, okay. Sorry. Thanks for getting back to me."

Let me repeat: in life, always take a thorough history *before* you make a judgment.

Exception to Every Rule

I talk about taking a good history, but as with every good rule, there are the unavoidable exceptions. Sometimes in emergency medicine, there is either no time or no opportunity to take a history: a one-day-old baby was found abandoned in a dumpster; a homeless person with no identification was hit by a car and remains unconscious. These things happen, sadly, all too often.

There were so many times when we had to assess what was wrong and speculate a lifetime of history—while also keeping all their vital signs going. We would search for any clues or physical signs to help us choose the correct drug, order the correct lab tests or imaging studies, or perform the correct procedures. This was all done under the pressure of knowing that if we made the wrong choice—if without our knowledge the person was allergic to a lifesaving medication—the consequences could be grave.

At the same time, there would always be the possibility that this individual was infected with a highly virulent organism capable of being transmitted to any or all of us who were in close contact. Plus, we had to be concerned about potential exposure to biochemical hazardous materials.

All of this had to occur within seconds to minutes, while we remained aware of the other patients already being treated and those coming in from the waiting room.

In order to accomplish all these things—practically simultaneously—we in emergency medicine used a lot of the same philosophy, rules, and application of protocols as the airlines do. To avoid mistakes, we utilized checklists and algorithms. Then we also had ways to evaluate any mistakes for improvement and to create assurances that we would learn something and not make a similar mistake in the future.

If you want to have a future, don't
do anything with no future in it.

—*Wu Cheng'en in* Journey to the West

Tales from the Trail: EeeeYahr

Sometimes there were unique shifts in the emergency department: the ones where everything went right—nothing went wrong. Those were good shifts.

But when everything went right, *and* you got the makings of a good story? That, my friends, was a *special* shift!

One of the greatest things about working in the ED was when the doctors got together and started swapping stories—each trying to outdo the other.

On one particularly fun day in my life, one of the head writers for a new television show called *ER* came to Santa Barbara. He was a friend of one of the emergency doctors in town, so about ten of us were invited to meet at the doctor's home with the writer. We spent almost twelve hours telling one story after another, each of us reliving and enjoying all the tales. From this event, many of the plots and subplots for the series were born.

As an aside, I could never watch that very popular show because I would get too involved. If the doctor didn't get the diagnosis fast enough or (worse yet) missed the diagnosis completely, I would start yelling at the TV screen! If they gave the wrong medicine, I would get even louder! Watching that show was more stressful than working a shift.

But here are a couple of good stories that come to mind:

It's a Miracle!

A nursing-home patient was sent to the hospital for a full workup. After the doctors and lab techs finished the examinations and tests, the nurses got the patient out of bed to walk in an effort to make sure the person could go back to the nursing home.

THE PATH OF LEAST EXISTENCE

Nobody is released from the hospital if they can't get up and walk. It took three nurses and two techs to get the patient up and walking—albeit with only slight success. But at that point, a nurse went outside to tell the nursing home's driver that the patient was able to walk and was ready to be discharged.

The driver stated, "That's amazing because that patient hasn't walked for over twenty years."

Smith & Wesson and Rolex

It was a typical Saturday evening at our little hospital in Beverly Hills, California. And when I say "typical" in an emergency department, I mean there is nothing typical—everything is unique. You never know who is going to come in, with what, and why.

Meanwhile, in another part of the city, an older man was sitting in his mobile home when he heard a noise outside. He ran out to witness a young guy stealing his car. Even though the car was already out of the driveway and speeding down the street, the older man knew he had two advantages over the young guy: One, he was already moving quickly to retrieve—and use—his Smith & Wesson .38 revolver. And two, he also knew the car was headed in the direction of a cul-de-sac and would be forced to come past him again in a few moments.

In the hospital, our paramedic radio signal went off. As we were all conditioned to do, we came closer to the radio and perked our senses to get as much information as possible to prepare us for "the who and the what." "We're coming in Code 3 [lights and sirens] with a sixteen-year-old male with a GSW [gunshot wound] to the chest. Two large-bore IVs have been started, and the patient is in shock. At your back door in one minute."

With no time to think, I started giving directions to the team: "Prepare the trauma room, get me an intubation tray... and get me the chest tray. I may have to crack his chest. Get lab and X-ray here for a trauma panel, type and cross for two units of blood. I want a stat chest X-ray. And get a Foley [urinary catheter] in him. Notify the surgeon and the OR [operating room]."

By this time, the entire team all had high adrenaline levels. We were very focused and coming together as an orchestra. Clerks were making calls, nurses and techs were getting equipment together, and I was preparing to do my initial assessment.

The young man lay undressed and unconscious on the trauma table. His breathing was labored and shallow, and his pulse was weak, irregular, and fading. I immediately intubated him, placing a large tube down his trachea (windpipe), and we began to control his breathing (which also helped me control my own breathing).

I next focused on the chest. Blood was coming out of the entrance wound—around the size of a .38-caliber bullet. It was about two inches to the right of his sternum (breastbone) and about two inches below his right clavicle (collarbone). I also noted that the right side of his chest was not rising when the respiratory therapist was bagging him. I checked and made sure the endotracheal tube was in the right place. It was.

That meant that he probably had a collapsed lung, and blood was filling up his chest. I checked his back, and there was no exit wound. An X-ray was placed on the view box, and I saw the bullet lodged in his chest. The surgeon had not yet arrived, and in my mind, this patient had only one chance for life.

I opened the chest tray and put a tube in his chest. Blood came pouring out through the tube, covering both my scrubs and those of the nurse standing next to me. The heart monitor revealed a slowing heart, near a flat line. I decided to open his chest.

I sterilized the chest, surgically draped the area, anesthetized the site, placed the scalpel between the fourth and fifth ribs anteriorly on the right... and opened his chest. He remained unconscious. I was on his right side; my head was near his face where the breathing tube was taped to his right cheek. My right hand was exploring his chest cavity for the bleeding blood vessel.

I couldn't see well because of all the blood, so I relied on my sense of feel. At this moment, three amazing things happened: (1) I found the bleeding vessel. (2) I found the bullet. (3) The young man sat upright with his eyes wide open.

As he sat up, my body, head, and arm moved with him. We stared at each other for an eternity—probably only a fraction of a second—while my right hand was still inside his chest holding the blood vessel and the bullet.

Everyone witnessed it, and there were gasps from all around the room. His body and head went back down again. None of us had time to respond to what we'd just witnessed. But I still envision it years later.

The surgeon came in, took the patient to the OR, and worked on him all night. They were still in surgery when morning arrived. I finished my shift, but I knew I was coming back that night and would find out what happened. Even though the patient had committed a crime, I put that aside *and wished him well.*

I started my next evening shift at 19:00 (7:00 p.m.). It was another busy night. But I found out from the nursing staff, the patient was alive—extubated in the ICU (intensive care unit). He was stable and improving. The emergency department quieted down around midnight, and I finally made my way to the ICU to see him. As I entered his room, I felt a little smile come over me, mentally patting myself on the back, knowing we saved his life. It was a great save by a great team.

"Hi. My name is Dr. Wollman. I was the doctor in the emergency department last night when you came in by ambulance."

He looked up at me and without hesitation asked, "Are you the one who stole my Rolex?"

Animal Antics

It was in a small, rural emergency department on the Central Coast of California—farm, horse, and wine country. I was the medical director, working a day shift.

This classic "story" day started with my very first patient, a tourist visiting an emu farm. Chief complaint: being pecked by an emu and receiving a large laceration to the face. Luckily, it wasn't very busy in this little hospital, so I had time to converse with the man while suturing his face back together (satisfying the desire I once had to be a plastic surgeon).

It took about an hour, and we had some good laughs about the story he was going to tell his friends when he returned from vacation. In my mind, I was already conjuring up my own version.

Then the second patient of the day, also a tourist, arrived by rental car. Chief complaint: head-butted by a llama at the nearby llama ranch. He had a large, bleeding laceration to his scalp. While suturing his laceration, we all laughed and worked on *his* story.

It didn't matter what happened for the rest of the shift. This was a great day!

But it was about to get better.

Patient Three arrived by ambulance. He was a cowboy who lived and worked on his nearby ranch. Chief complaint: chest and back pain after being "butt-butted" (is that even a term?) by a cow.

Simply stated—and without understanding bovine flirtations—the cow had backed her butt up against a fence with the cowboy, unfortunately, crushed in between.

He ended up with multiple, nondisplaced rib fractures, but otherwise he was fine. As word spread throughout the hospital, more and more personnel came in to hear the story. He continued to humorously describe the incident so our staff could picture it in great detail. Each time he laughed, the rib pain forced him to clutch his chest, but it never stopped him from coming up with increasingly embellished renditions.

Patients Four and Five came together in the family car. Chief complaint of Patient Four, a young boy: accidentally choked by a dog leash while in the backseat of the car.

Patient Five's chief complaint: no verbal complaint. Because Patient Five was the dog... who was on the leash... who had jumped out of the moving car... and was running alongside... but couldn't run quite as fast as the car... causing tension on the leash, which had accidentally wrapped around the neck of Patient Four.

Both were fine (although the dog had some minor abrasions to his foot pads).

As my shift of twelve hours was nearing its end, I was lying down in the on-call room, reflecting on the day and how superb it had been. The phone rang, and it was the ED calling for me to see a patient.

She arrived by ambulance from a local large-animal veterinarian's office. Chief complaints: kicked in the chest by a horse, and an extensive bite to the forearm. Both happened while she was assisting the vet. The horse kicked her to the ground, bit down, vise-like, on her forearm, and proceeded to rear his head—lifting her off the ground.

It turns out some horses just don't take kindly to being castrated!

It really was a special shift.

I love emergency medicine. (Can you tell?)

Chapter Twelve

I Feel My Pain (and It Helps Me Understand Yours)

I've observed and treated people with various illnesses and the chronic suffering involved. I feel fortunate that in my life, I have had very few illnesses.

On the other hand, I have had perhaps more than my share of injuries and pain, both acute and chronic.

As you would imagine, in the emergency department many patients would arrive in severe pain—say, from a hip injury. At times, some would say, "You have no idea how bad this is, and how much it hurts!"

I would quietly reflect to myself, "Oh, but I do. I really, really do."

I am essentially in pain every day but grateful that it isn't worse than it is. I'm grateful I am able to function and enjoy life, grateful for the many things that don't hurt, and grateful for the moments when the pain is gone. Sometimes, I feel the pain as if it's a shadow, and on a few occasions, I feel it as if it's a ghost. Those are pretty good moments. I can feel the pain trying to connect with me, but I am slightly, carefully, ahead of it.

But every morning as I prepare to get out of bed, I am immediately hit with the same, sobering concerns. What is going to happen when I put my foot down on the floor? Will my joints support my weight today, or will I crumble into a heap and require assistance? Will I be able to manage the pain, or is today going to be "one of those days"?

Every. Single. Day.

Pain in the...

So, let's back up. What caused my pain? "Let me count the ways."

Don't worry, I don't feel the need to chronicle the "trauma" of my birth. We all did that! My circumcision wasn't particularly noteworthy—at least for the purpose of this discussion. (Although I can assure you it was noteworthy to me.)

I had my tonsils and adenoids removed as a youth, but those were very popular surgeries in my era. I lived through the then-common childhood diseases (measles, mumps, chicken pox, and even German measles while in college).

I had the typical tooth extractions required for braces, and later wisdom teeth extractions and root canals as well. Probably you have too.

I'm even of the age now to have experienced bilateral cataract surgery and bilateral lens implants (allowing me, one might say, to look at life through new lenses). But even though I learned from all those experiences, none of them resulted in unusual or long-lasting pain.

However, starting around age ten, I developed ingrown toenails. My doctor established a plan: every day soak my feet in hot, nearly boiling water with Epsom salts, followed by monthly painful digging with a scalpel to open the area. Three surgeries and forty-five years later, that issue was finally resolved. (Well, except for the surgical absence of one great toenail.)

Cane but Able

I mentioned earlier that I started walking very early, but due to a serious injury sustained to my right hip while playing college intramural football at age nineteen, I began walking with a cane, "gutting it out," thus moving through my undergrad years in pain.

No one could figure out what was wrong. There were many theories, tentative diagnoses, and a myriad of potential solutions (such as "no weight-bearing for a year," and then we would see what might happen; um, that's not going to happen!).

The pain was getting worse and more persistent as I entered medical school. In my third year of medical school, as I was doing a rotation through orthopedic surgery, I met Augusto Sarmiento, MD—Professor and Chairman Emeritus (Orthopedics), University of Miami; later, Director of Orthopedics, Orthopedic Hospital, and Professor and Chairman of Orthopedics, University of Southern California.

I saw him for a consult about my relentless hip pain and frustration regarding the lack of a definitive diagnosis. He ordered an X-ray of my pelvis that finally showed the problem. At the ripe young age of twenty-two, I had the hip of an eighty-five-year-old man!

I finally had a diagnosis: aseptic necrosis of the head of my right femur. I had lost the blood supply to the head of the femur, and it had died.

I immediately reflected back to a day in college at the University of Florida, three days after my football injury. I felt an electrical jolt that began in my right hip and instantly went through my entire body. I remember it happened when I was walking down some stairs to get from one class to another. It was so bad that it abruptly straightened my entire body, and I almost fell down the stairs.

Looking back, I believe that was the moment of the death of my femoral head.

But I digress.

I didn't realize my good fortune at the time, or how that same good fortune would return multiple times in my life. Sir John Charnley, CBE, FRS (a British orthopedic surgeon), pioneered the total hip replacement procedure. Today, it is one of the most common operations both in the UK and elsewhere in the world, but at the time, it was brand new.

Dr. Sarmiento was one of the early pioneers in the United States, and he was at my medical school. I remember looking at him across his desk as he sat with the glaring X-ray behind him. I had mixed emotions: I was happy to finally receive a diagnosis and a potential cure, but I was mourning the fact that I had such an old, painful hip. I suppose one psychological benefit of this injury was that I experienced my midlife crisis at a very early age.

I said, "Let's do the surgery."

He said, "No."

Limping on My Path

As I mentioned, at this time the hip replacement procedure was very new; they were just learning about and perfecting it. So, at this point they only operated on overweight, elderly, arthritic people with limited activity. That way, by working with people who were not too active, they could more precisely document semi-long-term results and complications. A twenty-two-year-old medical student with an entire life ahead of him did not fit their constraints.

Frustrated and depressed, I immediately came up with a plan: I would go straight through my last two years of med school without vacation, finish a few months early, speak with Dr. Sarmiento again, have the surgery in April of 1972, and heal before starting an internship in June.

After limping through those last two years, I approached Dr. Sarmiento again. This time, I changed my strategy. I said, "I have wanted to be a doctor my whole life. I'm finishing medical school early with the hope that you will now agree to do the surgery. If you don't, I will not be in any condition to do an internship or residency, much less practice medicine!"

I will never forget as he pondered for a few moments, then said, "Let's do it!"

I was back on track.

He operated. I graduated, walking across the stage on crutches to receive my MD degree. I flew out to California in the fall of 1972 and continued to follow my path—albeit with a limp for the rest of my life.

Fortunately for me, Dr. Sarmiento eventually moved to Los Angeles as well, to take a position at USC Orthopedic Hospital. He reentered and repaired my hip and pelvis on two more occasions, once following an accident and later because of a potential tumor.

I will forever be grateful to him. Because of his knowledge and expertise, I was able to stay on my path.

The Eyes Have It

In the second year of my surgical residency, I was tasked with doing a pre-op exam on a patient scheduled for an inguinal hernia repair.

As part of the complete exam, I used an ophthalmoscope to examine the internal parts of the patient's eyes. The procedure is to hold the instrument in your right hand, use your right eye to examine the patient's right eye, and then do the exact opposite for the left eye.

I was surprised to see that the patient was completely missing the important anatomical parts for vision in his right eye. There was no history of vision impairment, and he clearly had seen me walk in the room.

I immediately checked his left eye, and again, I could not see his optic nerve or any normal blood vessels. With all this missing anatomy, there was no way he should have been able to see me.

What was going on?

I finally figured out that it was *my* vision that was suddenly impaired.

I consulted with an ophthalmologist on staff. He observed that something was wrong with both of my maculae but wasn't sure what it was. His suggestion was to either take steroids, which would help if the problem was an allergy, or completely avoid steroids, a tactic that could exacerbate the condition if it was caused by a virus. Either way, we would have to wait and see what happened.

I chose to avoid steroids.

When I tried to read with one eye closed, many of the words were missing. The lines of print would float upward when I used one eye and downward when I used the other. It was almost as if the exact opposite pathology was occurring in each eye so that when I used them together, the line would straighten out.

I consulted with two of the top eye centers in the country. No one knew what was wrong. In fact, they didn't even have a name for it. They created the provisional name "bilateral multifocal placoid epitheliopathy," but they had no treatment plan nor any idea of how it might progress.

The symptoms seemed to go away partially after a few months, but they returned again the following spring, causing some to surmise it could be a seasonal viral or allergic reaction. (Maybe I should have taken steroids.)

The condition continued to progress over my lifetime until a few years ago, when it seemed to have stabilized.

By the way, they finally did come up with a name for it (or the closest thing to it): Best disease. I guess I should consider that as small compensation for losing a portion of my central vision: I have a "best" disease. (I always was an overachiever.)

I have lived my entire adult life with the looming possibility that at any moment, I could go blind. That awareness makes me appreciate everything I do see and inspires admiration for those without vision.

My retinal specialist tells me that perhaps within the next few years, they might perfect a stem cell product that could be injected into my eyes, and they will be fixed. I will then be faced with the dichotomy of gaining good vision but losing the "best" disease.

What would your vote be? For me, the eyes have it.

Potholes

Years later, despite knowing better and as an ED doctor who treated many of those injured in the activity, I started riding a motorcycle. Feel free to insert your eye roll here, but I loved it! Until the afternoon of January 8, 1982, when I crashed and burned.

I sustained facial lacerations, leg burns, and multiple fractures. A pelvic fracture and accompanying hip prosthesis damage resulted in a complex surgical repair. My left wrist fracture and left elbow fracture required multiple surgeries to allow me to regain a functional left hand so that I could continue to practice medicine. In comparison to all these, the ankle fracture I also had seemed tame!

I was in the hospital for almost two months seriously resembling the proverbial cartoon with pins through two parts of my left arm, elevated on a pulley system, and pins in my elevated right leg, also attached to a pulley system. If it hadn't been so painful, it might have been funny.

I was grateful to all the doctors, nurses, physical therapists, family, and friends who got me through this ordeal. I remember, from my narcotic-induced state, feeling very depressed—considering death as a really good option—crying with tears rolling down my cheeks into my mouth. That's when I came up with this little ditty: "You don't know your fears till you've tasted your tears."

I thought I'd paid my dues. But apparently, I wasn't finished.

In 1984, I had a vasectomy. (Okay, that one I signed up for.) But meanwhile, it was discovered that I had hepatitis C (probably as a result of the multiple blood transfusions required during my earlier hip surgery). In 1992, I had another hip surgery to remove a benign tumor. A few years later, I had a herniated cervical spine disc repair performed (with fusion), followed quickly by a herniated lumbar spine disc repair as well.

I've battled trigeminal neuralgia (extremely severe nerve pain in the face and jaw) and temporomandibular joint pain (TMJ). I've had multiple cystoscopies for seemingly never-ending kidney stones, as well as a surgery to pulverize and retrieve a stone that was lodged in my urethra. I had another surgery to correct a ureter abnormality. And I know the pain of the self-urethral catheterizations that were necessary before my laser surgery for an enlarged prostate.

So, yes, I have felt pain. I've also managed to learn a few things from these experiences. First and foremost: Pain hurts! (Pretty original, huh?) But my experience—my personal understanding of the severity of pain—has molded me into an extremely empathetic doctor. For that, I and all of my patients are grateful.

I've also learned that living an active life, one sometimes on the edge, can cause injuries. Hopefully, this realization has made me less judgmental than some health-care practitioners who might prescribe living in bubble wrap to avoid trauma.

Working while in pain has taught me that either I have to deal with it, or it will deal with me. Who's in charge? I always try to retain the upper hand, but sometimes I can't. That helps me empathize.

Lastly, I have become an expert at "recovery." That has become a very important part of my medical practice. Most surgeons will tell you you're recovered much earlier than you actually are. I know the truth because I have lived it... over and over and over.

But none of these experiences compared to the painful events of my horrific car accident on 03/30/03.

 If you or a loved one is faced with a decision to undergo surgery, I encourage you to visit **GlennWollman.com/resources** and check out Guidepost 12—Roadside Service: The Surgical Suite.

Chapter Thirteen

All Roads Lead to the Medical Guide

Where your talents and the needs of the world cross, there lies your vocation.

—Aristotle

Inevitably, people have always asked me what I do. When they find out I am a doctor, the next question is "What is your specialty?"

After years of happily saying, "Emergency medicine," at my first opportunity to try out my new title, I told an inquiring gentleman that I was a Medical Guide.

I noticed he appeared perplexed as he asked, "What is a Medical God?"

So, apparently, in addition to actually designing what I would be doing as a Medical Guide, I also had to figure out how to pronounce it more clearly!

So, what is a Medical Guide? Here's my elevator pitch:

As a physician, I have practiced in the specialty of emergency medicine for over thirty years where humanity and health care intersect—and sometimes collide. Educated in both Western and integrative medicine, along with firsthand experience on both sides of the surgeon's scalpel, I know—and appreciate— the importance of informed medical decisions. I, therefore, created a specialized area in medicine.

I am a Medical Guide.

I provide support and knowledge to help my clients gain control of their health. I assist people in making difficult medical decisions through a holistic and integrative approach geared toward each individual's specific needs.

I assist in making a correct diagnosis and selecting the right team of health-care providers, and work with them to evaluate treatment options that reflect the best in Western practices, combining integrative practices when appropriate.

Through extensive communication with my client, I formulate a personalized plan that will not only address the medical issues at hand, but also analyze and balance crucial aspects of their lifestyle. This will help to identify potential factors that may have contributed to the current clinical dilemma and, most importantly, provide a path to healing and future optimal health.

To prevent complications from a procedure or avoid bad side effects from a treatment, I focus not only on the big decisions, such as surgery, radiation, or chemotherapy, but also on the day-to-day choices that have the potential to make life miserable.

Confusing health issues and an unfamiliar medical landscape can be intimidating. I know the territory, and I speak the language. I collaborate with my client, charting a path through diagnosis, treatment, recovery, and ongoing wellness.

When medical specialists come down with an injury or illness—even in their own specialty—they usually go to another physician to help make the critical decisions.

To avoid the stress of making wrong choices leading to perhaps avoidable catastrophe, consider consulting with and depending on a Medical Guide. Although this area of expertise isn't yet a specialty, try to find others to assist you on your journey. Try using search terms like *medical decision support*, *health care advocacy*, *health care navigation*, *patient care assistant*, or *patient navigator*. This would be a place to start, with the hope that someday soon these searches will also include the other multitude of healing modalities from around the globe, woven into Western medicine. Know that because "Medical Guide" isn't a medical specialty (as yet), there's no one search term that would pull up exactly what I do, but we must start somewhere. My hope is that if you're interested in a career in helping others attain optimal health, you would consider becoming a Medical Guide and helping the field become a regulated specialty that would include the areas I describe in this book.

Pragmatically Speaking

So, how does that work in practice? Let's start from the first and most obvious starting point—the one we are most familiar with: making medical decisions after we get sick or injured.

Say you have pain in your right lower abdomen with vomiting. Your doctor says, "You're having an appendicitis attack, and you need a surgeon to take out your inflamed appendix."

Not much medical guidance is really necessary, right?

On the other hand, if you develop a rare tumor or a complicated illness and you receive multiple and possibly contradictory opinions, this is a good time for a Medical Guide. As the name implies, he or she is there to guide you through the confusion when the direction is not clear.

For the purpose of explanation, let's say you break your forearm. One orthopedic surgeon tells you that pins, screws, plates, and all sorts of hardware are necessary for a good repair and healing.

You're very nervous about the surgery, so you go to another orthopedic surgeon for a second opinion. She tells you that it will heal fine in a cast without any surgery! This course of action sounds much more appealing, but you are paralyzed by uncertainty because you were previously told you could properly heal only with all the hardware.

What to do?

Search for a Medical Guide who will use science to help analyze the type of fracture and combine that with an in-depth knowledge of your general health. The guide will determine whether you are a diabetic with poor healing qualities and will factor in your eventual needs and desires for a specific outcome. The guide will determine whether you are a piano virtuoso requiring very fine dexterity in your hands and fingers or a grape stomper requiring more dexterity in your toes and feet.

At this point you might be asking, "Why would this be any different than any other medical consultation?"

I commend you on the question, and here is the answer:

Your Medical Guide will escort you to the decision that best fits with your own personal needs. All of the consultations and opinions may be correct for one reason or another. There may even be additional alternatives to your condition that have not yet been suggested. But only one of these courses of action may be the best fit.

Also, if required, a Medical Guide will determine how best to prepare your body and mind for a procedure and the subsequent healing process. It is likely your guide will offer a combination of Western allopathic medicine with an alternative medicine, such as acupuncture or Ayurvedic medicine—what I call combinatorial medicine.

On a practical level, when illness strikes, a Medical Guide can determine whether you require an immediate trip to the urgent care center or the emergency department.

If your condition is not emergent, your guide can prepare you for a regularly scheduled doctor's appointment. Your primary care doctor may not have sufficient time to answer all your questions, but your guide can further educate you on your diagnosis. When necessary, they can also facilitate a consult with a specialist in another part of the country (or in another country entirely). They can also serve the vital function of counseling your close family members, relatives, and friends to allay their concerns or fears.

Medical Guides many times provide for improved healing because they possess an overview of all your interactions with various specialists and can remove redundancies. By utilizing a combinatorial approach, lowering doses of certain medications and possibly eliminating other medications entirely may translate to fewer side effects.

 To learn six different ways of making decisions, visit **GlennWollman.com/resources** and check out Guidepost 1—Navigation: Spooning the Fork in the Road.

Preparatory Medicine

Finally, on a deeper level, a Medical Guide can assist with what I consider one of the most important aspects of health care in the twenty-first century: staying healthy by keeping a balanced life.

Certainly, Western medicine has done a great service to humanity in healing the sick—especially in emergency and critical care, my area of expertise. But historically, we've focused only on *preventing* sickness and ills in the areas of immunizations and foreign travel (such as antimalarial medications).

In general, the public has accepted this pattern—until the end of the last century, when alternative medicines entered the mainstream. We began taking vitamins and supplements to keep ourselves healthy. People also began to exercise more to either become or stay fit.

This is a good thing. This is all to prevent disease and injury. But it is now time to move to the next phase: to live a balanced life exclusively for the sake of the balanced life itself and not merely for the prevention of something sinister.

Ergo, I offer the concept of "preparatory medicine." This concept differs from preventive medicine. You can't prevent everything, but you most assuredly can prepare by living in the best possible health in body, mind, and spirit. Frankly, it only makes logical sense to be in the best condition possible at all times because that, in itself, may prevent certain illnesses and injuries. But in case the unavoidable does occur, your existence in optimum balance will help you mentally through the incident and will also bolster healing.

This requires a careful analysis of specific categories that have been shown to affect the immune system and other physiological systems that the body uses for prevention of infections, inflammation, allergic reactions, and bleeding.

These categories are what I have termed the Six Aspects of Optimal Health. They inform Our Path.

 For a quick checklist to help bring more awareness to your physical fitness, visit **GlennWollman.com/ resources** and check out Guidepost 13—Watch the Road Signs: Slow Down Ahead.

The doctor of the future will give no medication but will interest his patients in the care of the human frame, in diet, and in the cause and prevention of disease.

— *Thomas Alva Edison*

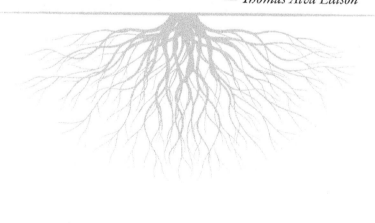

PART TWO

Everyone's Path:
Six Aspects of Optimal Health

Chapter Fourteen

"Helllllo, Aspects!"

Throughout my practice, my primary focus in medicine has been a correct diagnosis and an appropriate treatment. Makes sense, right?

Secondly, I delve deeply for cause and effect. In my specialty, I had great opportunities to see humanity in varying degrees of crisis mode—from birth to death and everything in between.

What stood out to me was that certain people handled their situations with ease, and others couldn't handle crises at all; certain people healed well, and others healed poorly; certain people died well, and others died poorly.

I yearned to discover factors that would improve the odds—factors I could apply to both myself and others. Eventually, I was able to identify Six Aspects that unquestionably make a difference.

Some of this is not new. Over time, science—and the medical world—have come to recognize these as "lifestyle changes." Everyone now agrees that sound Nutrition and Physical Activity are vital. More recently, both Sleep Management and Stress Management have been added to newly trending lifestyle medicine programs.

For those of you counting, yes, we are at four, and I know you are begging, "Please, please, Glenn. Tell us the other two. We want... no, we *need* to know!"

Well, just for you, the two other factors that I hope eventually will be widely recognized are **Spirituality** and **Patterns of Behavior**.

Now that you are aware of these six factors—the Six Aspects of Optimal Health—the next important thing to do is address them. And by "address," I don't mean Art Carney's old comedy routine, "Helllllllo, Aspects!" No. I mean that you have to move them from intellect to consciousness. You can't just know about them; they need to be established as a conscious practice on a daily basis.

For example, you can't just "know" the Surgeon General's warning on a package of cigarettes and yet continue to smoke. That is stopping at mere intellect. You must appreciate the myriad effects smoking has on body, mind, and spirit, and consciously make a change for the sake of optimal health.

Addressing one, two, or even three of these aspects is certainly beneficial, but if you don't address all six, you have almost no chance at true optimal health. If you eat well and exercise like a triathlete, that is good, but if at the same time, you sleep poorly and are always stressed...

Well, you know what I'm getting at, and I hope you see the point.

It's about the balance of each of the Six Aspects of Optimal Health. The body, mind, and spirit are interconnected. If one is out of alignment, all aspects are affected. Being out of balance is manifested in many ways: physical and mental illness, difficulty in personal and professional relationships, career frustration, and loss of general well-being.

Balance is the key—in everything. One of my brothers taught me two important things based on his experience as a 747 pilot.

His philosophical view:

Whether you view the tank as half empty or half full, it takes you the same distance.

His political view:
You need a left and a right wing to fly somewhere.
He was advocating simple and logical balance.

The Environment

Even with balance and doing all the right things, the environment around you plays an integral part in your overall health. Viruses, bacteria, fungi, parasites, toxins, and pollutants are a few of the environmental hazards you can't always dodge.

An example? Plastic waste.

When I was a kid, Plastic Man was my favorite comic book superhero. His superpower? The ability to morph into any object. I'm not sure what intrigued me more: my desire to have the stealth of that power myself or the fact that his head and his red uniform always remained as tell-tale elements of the object he became (tell-tale signs that none of the bad guys ever seemed to notice).

Currently, we know that because of the sheer volume of plastic that has been used and then disposed of over the years, there is an unbelievable amount in landfills and our oceans. Scientists have discovered it in our tap and bottled water and currently are finding particles in the air we breathe... even in the most remote areas of the planet!

Because nature cannot break them down quickly, microplastic particles have become part of our environment. These particles have found their way into birds, fish, shellfish, and mammals. It is therefore obvious that small, microscopic plastics are found in human bodies. By the time you read this, we will be developing names for the various syndromes caused by these plastics.

What are the long-term effects of microscopic plastics in our system? What microorganisms might attach to the plastics as they enter our system? Could they be contributors to blocked arteries? Are they contributing to diseases? Are they avoidable, or have we assaulted our environment to the point of no return?

As a kid, I wanted to be Plastic Man, and now I very well may be becoming him. Unfortunately, it doesn't feel like a superpower.

A Brief Introduction to Your Body: Cell Mates

Before we get ahead of ourselves and move through the Six Aspects, let's move backward (or should I say, inward). Your body is made up of systems, such as the digestive system and the skeletal system. Each system is made of organs, such as the stomach and the femur. Each organ is made of tissues. And eventually, we get to our individual cells. We will refer back to the remarkable cell on many occasions in this book, because *that is where the action is.*

Our bodies consist of more than thirty-seven trillion cells. Each one is made up of specific structures and has specific functions: one is to survive and duplicate in order to produce other cells, and the second is to perform a particular function; e.g., muscle cells perform contraction and blood cells carry oxygen and nutrients to other cells.

Think of it this way: You don't have a lung; you have lung cells working together to create what we recognize as a lung. When you take a deep breath, you are actually delivering oxygen into the myriad lung cells that collectively make up what you call your lung. You are filling cells with oxygen.

You are affecting your body on a cellular level with every involuntary and voluntary decision you make. It's an important distinction that will change the way you perceive and care for your body and your cells.

While eating a chocolate cake, you have probably always thought you are merely sending a delicious chocolate cake to your stomach.

You are not.

You are sending macro- and micronutrients—sugar, caffeine, saturated fat, sodium, and so on—to a group of stomach cells. You are asking those *cells* to break down and assimilate these molecular ingredients—determine what is waste, what is nutritious, and what is toxic—and pass each component through to other specific cells that will in turn perform their functions.

When your cells are reproducing or repairing themselves, they rely on the nutrients you deliver to them. Are you using a Twinkie as fuel while your brain cells are making repairs?

When you start thinking on a cellular level, you will think more carefully about what you ingest. Note: If you have a Twinkie in your hand as you are reading this, skip to the chapter on nutrition. You'll need it sooner rather than later!

Equally important are the mitochondria within the cells. The mitochondria are the parts of the cell that use the nutrients we consume to create energy in order for the cell to function. As we age and get exposed to toxins and free radicals, the mitochondria degrade and become less effective. This can cause inflammation and cell mutations. For a long, healthy life, the best plan is to protect the mitochondria through a balance of the Six Aspects of Optimal Health.

(A small prediction for the future of physical fitness: it is not just the size of our muscles; it is the number of mitochondria within the muscle cells that makes the muscle most effective. Right now, as we exercise, we unknowingly create more mitochondria to make bigger and more effective musculature.)

Oh, and there is one more place in your body where things happen: within the organisms living inside of you. Yes, there is more inside of you that *isn't* you than there is *of* you. In case you didn't quite get that, let me repeat: there is more genetic material in your body belonging to bacteria, viruses, fungi, and other little creatures than there is of your *own* genetic material. We are basically hosting them until we die.

Some of these creatures in your body are kept at bay by your immune system. Coincidentally, much of your immune system is made up of beneficial organisms living inside your body—a high percentage of them living in your intestinal tract. When your immune system is compromised, the opportunistic creatures wreak havoc—creatures such as the herpes zoster virus (causing shingles), the *Neisseria meningitidis* bacteria (causing meningococcal meningitis), or the *Pneumocystis carinii/jirovecii* fungus (causing a form of pneumonia), just to name a few.

If such organisms were left unfettered, our corpses would serve as a banquet for these hitchhikers until there was nothing left of us. So, aside from protecting and loving your own cells, you must protect all the good organisms that keep the opportunistic pathogens away—or the bad guys will start digesting you before you are finished hosting.

Simply said, as you approach the trailhead of your path of health, put this reminder message in your travel bag: cellular health is the basis of optimal health.

The Sum of All Parts or Some of the Parts

If you are still living in the nineteenth or twentieth century, I would like to suggest that you purchase an anatomy book. There are so many out there, telling you which one to buy would not be as beneficial as telling you to do some research and find the one that fits you best. Make sure it is one that has plenty of easy-to-understand pictures and descriptions.

If you are in the twenty-first century, get a good anatomy app or program on one of your electronic devices. They're starting to teach anatomy with holograms now. It shouldn't be long before it comes free with your phone (but that doesn't mean you should wait for it to come out).

So, for now, having an anatomy app or book will give you great power to gain some understanding of your physical body.

This does not mean you have to become an anatomy professor or a surgeon, but understanding where things are and where things connect will give you some idea of your body's function. All of this will come in handy when I discuss diagnosis and mechanism of injury further along in this book.

Understanding anatomy will also help you decide how to treat an injury (whether your own or a family member's or a friend's). It will surely assist in making the determination whether or not to see a doctor or go to an emergency department. And it will give you a sense of power. If you believe that doctors believe they are gods, you, too, can share in the power.

Owning an anatomy book can be a clever way to interest your children in their bodies and help them become less scared of blood and guts and more knowledgeable about illness or injury.

And now (drumroll, please), the best reason to have an understanding of anatomy, and one of the great things I loved about medical training: you very well might develop a better appreciation for your body. Because of that newfound appreciation, you will possibly—and I say only "possibly"— take care of it a little more and have gratitude for all the parts that are working well even if you have one part that might be in a state of dysfunction.

Chapter Fifteen

The Goldilocks Strategy

Life is like riding a bicycle. To keep your balance, you must keep moving.

—*Albert Einstein*

Also understand that while we may think we should endeavor for perfection, actually achieving perfection is neither possible nor necessarily desirable.

Take a page from Goldilocks' experience as you incorporate each of the following Six Aspects of Optimal Health. Attempt to strike a balance that is "*juuuuuust right.*"

It's the 80/20 rule. Figure out how good your habits are in each aspect, and then slowly try to improve to 80 percent good habits and only 20 percent not so good. This allows for the slow, effective adaptations to our behavior that are necessary for most of us to change successfully. Over time, as it becomes easier, you may naturally move to higher percentages: 85 percent, 90 percent, 95 percent. You never have to get to 100 percent. Get real.

Chapter Sixteen

PATTERNS OF BEHAVIOR:
Lather, Rinse, Repeat

Before you heal someone, ask him if he is willing to give up the things that made him sick.

—*Hippocrates*

Sink-chronicity

Each time we start and end a shift, serious information needs to be transmitted from the outgoing doctor to the incoming doctor. First and foremost, an immediate picture of "Here's what I'm leaving you" must be painted. The brush strokes are the current situation in staffing, on-call issues, inpatient bed availability, etc. Then we introduce the painting's subjects—the patients: what stage of diagnosis and treatment each is in, and whether there are life-threatening situations. (Although, I must say, when there is an ongoing life-threatening situation, the incoming doctor will usually be tipped off by a lot of blood, instruments, machines, and a high level of energy in the form of controlled chaos.)

Once the serious information is transmitted with confidence, if time and patients permit, then the entertaining stories and tales are shared. (I explain this because I can claim as true only the experiences in which I have been personally involved. This one was told to me, but I thought it was worth retelling. At the time this story was told, the patient was no longer in the department. And for privacy, I will refer to this person as genderless, simply "the patient.")

The patient, accompanied by frantic family members, appeared in the waiting room in a lot of pain. The right hand—wrapped with bloodied towels—was held in the air, being assisted by the left. At triage, the patient was immediately taken to a bed.

The injured hand was bloody with arterial "spurters." (I don't really think I need to explain that image, do I?) There were deep lacerations on the thumb, index, and middle fingers, with bone fragments and connective tissue appearing in the wound. It was obvious—in seconds—this was an emergency surgical case.

After the patient was stabilized, the assessment began. Getting the history, as always, started with the "chief complaint"—basically, "What brings you to our hospital at this time?"

In this case, it was obvious.

At this time, it was vital to assess whether there was nerve damage to the injured fingers (through motor function, sensation to light touch, pain, and two-point discrimination—testing the ability to sense whether two objects touching the skin are indeed two objects or just one). This assessment determines the type of specialist required to be called: an orthopedic surgeon, a hand specialist, and/or a neurosurgeon.

With the basic information established, then came the question of the cause of this mangling of skin, blood vessels, nerves, tendons, ligaments, and bones. We call this the "mechanism of injury."

The patient had accidentally dropped a sharp, serrated steak knife into the in-sink garbage disposal and, yep, you guessed it, reached in to get it while the motor was running.

(Okay, I'll let you take a moment to squeamishly imagine what it would feel like if it were *your* right hand—or left, for you lefties out there. I realize this is mind-boggling in and of itself. But wait—there's more!)

Even though there did not appear to be any current injury to the ring and pinky fingers, the doctor noticed loss of sensation in these two fingers as well. It made no sense to the astute and well-trained physician. This damage couldn't have happened during this incident because these fingers are on completely different nerve tracts.

He expressed his concern and confusion as to why these two seemingly undamaged fingers were not normal.

The patient quickly solved the mystery by explaining, "Oh, yeah, Doc! That's because I did this exact same thing a few years ago and injured *those* two fingers that time."

I've always said, stupid, clumsy, and angry gave us all job security in the emergency department. But, more importantly, this illustrates how difficult it is to change Patterns of Behavior.

We are constantly exhibiting our patterns—sometimes based on fact and sometimes based on myth. Some are beneficial (looking both ways before crossing the street; brushing your teeth after every meal; saying "please" and "thank you"). It is crucial, however, that we recognize the patterns that don't serve us well—and change them into better patterns. But it isn't always about removing a bad pattern. Perhaps at times we will need to add a new pattern that never existed.

Patterns of Behavior is easily the most important of the Six Aspects of Optimal Health. Mastering it informs how we tackle the remaining five aspects in order to make positive changes. Remember, our minds change at the speed of light. No, not at 186,000 miles per second. Minds change in the time it takes for you to see the light.

Fetal Hijinks: Pre- and Postnatal Patterns

Beginning in utero, physiological patterns regulating vital bodily functions develop in the deepest recesses of the brain. Functions such as breathing, heartbeat and heart rate, temperature control, and waking and sleeping cycles remain on a subconscious level throughout our lifetime. (Can you imagine if you had to think about and control each breath or heartbeat? There wouldn't be any time to play or eat.)

As the fetal brain and spinal cord grow, all the parts begin to make their connections. The spinal reflex, simple knee jerk, startle reflex, sucking reflex, and grasping reflex originate, among others.

With the developing brain busy working on the physiology, the fetal mind begins to establish Patterns of Behavior, also in utero, and continues throughout life. Whether Mommy-to-Be is feeling happy, stressed, or angry, hormones circulate. They eventually make their way to the little being in the uterus, and these hormones affect the developing cells. More and more patterns develop well before the baby's grand entrance (or exit, depending on your point of view).

The fun—and complications—begin when Mom, Dad, and a host of others start interacting with this new being. Mixed messages begin to tie knots in the baby's mind.

Soft, comforting, loving sounds and sensations are showered on the infant when their little hand reflexively wraps around the parent's finger for the first time. (This is, as you might recall, the grasping reflex I mentioned a few lines back.) The same wonderful feedback comes when the little developing hand grasps the baby rattle.

The message, although obviously without adequate vocabulary in this early stage, is "Good things happen when I put something between my fingers. Everyone around me seems to like it, and I get rewarded.

"I think I'll grab that sharp pencil.

"Wait! What are all those loud noises and anger and sharp slapping on my hand? I don't get it! Is it good or bad to put things in my cute little baby hand? I'm confused."

As we grow up, we receive many mixed messages, further developing our confusing patterns of behavior.

Early on, we develop patterns based on survival, especially in a dysfunctional family. You may not have full understanding of the things happening around you, but if your developing patterns keep you alive, then you retain them. While Mom and Dad are screaming at each other, locking yourself in your room, burying yourself in books, looking for somewhere to hide, or eating junk food can be your salvation. The problems form when you keep those patterns much longer than you need to— into adulthood, when you should have a better understanding of circumstances and can eliminate patterns that are no longer necessary.

My sister, attaining her doctoral degree in special education, realized her professional Mission was to care for kids with special needs and challenging patterns of behavior. She also spent a great deal of her family life rescuing animals mistreated by adults with very distorted and cruel patterns of behavior. Some of her influence made me realize the importance of this Aspect of Optimal Health.

Pattern Recognition 101

Okay, if you don't agree that you have established lifelong patterns of behavior, then follow me on a virtual trip to your bathroom—one of the easiest places to observe patterns.

Look at the way you put the toothpaste on your toothbrush, the way you brush your teeth, the way you wash and dry yourself in the shower (or maybe you prefer bath behavior). Watch how you get dressed, and in what order you put on clothing.

These are your patterns.

I could walk around with you all day long pointing out pattern after pattern. In fact, I urge you to think about your existing patterns as you go about your home, through your bedroom routine, as you cook and clean in your kitchen or get into your car. It's astounding how much of our behavior stems from well-established patterns.

Don't get me wrong; patterns in and of themselves are not bad! They are designed to make our lives easier, so we don't have to think about mundane things. We can spend more of our time enjoying ourselves or, as some seem to prefer, worrying about things that may never happen.

It is important to understand that we all have patterns of behavior. Sometimes you have to separate the person from their patterns. When someone acts badly or in an inappropriate manner, you don't have to accept or tolerate the bad behavior, but you can continue to love them. (It will make for a healthier and safer planet.)

So, here is the first step. Let's see how good you are at recognition, but more importantly, how capable or willing you are to change. Pick an inconsequential action like teeth brushing and observe your own pattern.

Then, for the sake of understanding, change the pattern! Start at the opposite side of your mouth or begin with the lower teeth rather than the upper.

How did that feel?

Teeth Flossing

My dentist told me that flossing is a good idea. It takes about eighteen hours for plaque-causing bacteria to grow, so it should be done at least once a day.

"Would it be a good idea, then, to floss twice a day? Around every twelve hours?" I asked.

He pondered the question, and then giggled, as though he had taken a hit of his nitrous oxide. "Yes," he said.

If you believe that flossing is a good idea, as an experiment, develop a new pattern of behavior to floss once when you awaken and then again before you go to sleep. Or, if you don't want to be quite that hard on yourself, merely attempt to change the order in which you floss the narrow crevices all the way to your illustrious gum line. If you aren't already a flosser, then perform the process once a day, as your new pattern of behavior. Commit to doing this for the rest of your life—or at least as long as you have teeth.

 For more tips on turning your bathroom into a place of Zen or simple observation, visit **GlennWollman. com/resources** and check out Guidepost 10—Pit Stop: Bathroom Work.

The 7 Keys to Modifying Pattern Behavior

1. First recognize and acknowledge that there is a problem.

2. Establish whether it is a pattern worth keeping or a pattern not beneficial to your health or happiness.

3. Direct your conscious will to change the pattern and analyze the benefits of changing it. (If you want to go Jungian, analyze why you developed the pattern in the first place.)

4. Come up with a few good choices for the new pattern and pick the best one, making sure it's something within your grasp.

5. Put the new pattern into effect.

6. Observe whether you continue the pattern and, more importantly, observe the times when you don't. Analyze the reasons for each. (This analysis will give you some clues to the subtler patterns— the conscious and subconscious reasons why you either can or can't change.)

7. Follow up often to ensure that the change remains and you haven't fallen back into the old pattern.

If you keep reverting, let that impress upon you how powerful patterns are—how much they want to control you and not let you change.

If, on the other hand, you recognized a pattern, changed it, and never looked back congratulations! You have just earned your first belt in the martial art of Pattern Changing!

Three other important things to note:

- You are the only one responsible for your patterns. It may be true that you developed a pattern at some point in response to someone else, but now that you are no longer a fetus, you can no longer blame your patterns of behavior on others.

- One tip for difficult change is to create a reward/ punishment system for success or failure. Allow yourself a treat if you remain consistent with your new Pattern of Behavior. (Although, actually, the beneficial result of the change should be enough reward in itself!) Conversely, assign a repercussion or ramification if you fall short in your initial attempts to change. (Perhaps let someone else know about this process, to keep yourself honest.)

- Most importantly, if you really want to change and can't, there is no need to go it alone. GET HELP from a friend or a professional.

There are important reasons your first attempt to change a pattern of behavior should be something as mundane as teeth flossing. Starting with simple patterns allows you to gain confidence. As you become more expert, you will begin to recognize, change, and maintain new patterns throughout your personal life and work.

For instance, when I read a chest X-ray, I have changed the customary Pattern of Behavior. I turn the X-ray upside down. This helps me see a different pattern than I am expecting, forcing me to look at it with a more discerning eye. (But it certainly took more effort to make this change than flossing twice a day.)

When you are ready, you will pick more difficult patterns with more consequences.

Mind Flossing

You've no doubt seen photos or drawings of the brain. If you bought your anatomy book or an app as I suggested earlier, check out all the nooks and crannies—the sulci and gyri—of the brain. If you think of them as places to hide within the brain, it becomes easier to imagine all the hiding places in your mind!

Sometimes you have patterns that might not be beneficial, but they are subtle in their ways. They're hiding. Mentally floss between the cracks and crevices of ideas and thoughts. Get between the conflicting and hidden thoughts, the long-forgotten reasons for a pattern. Floss them out. Expose hidden issues and, therefore, prevent mental "decay."

For instance, I have seen this scenario often—I'm sure you've seen it at least once as well. A woman marries a guy who turns out to be an alcoholic and wife beater. Amazingly, she eventually divorces him and marries another alcoholic and wife beater. And the beat goes on. She is caught in a loop pattern—a harmful loop pattern.

If you find yourself attracted to the wrong guys, time to mind floss.

Set aside a time during the day strictly for your mental flossing. Follow the same steps you successfully employed to change your pattern of teeth flossing.

But be careful. You might feel something hidden shooting out of a crevice, giving positive feedback of a "successful floss." Beware of cul-de-sacs, dead ends, coral reefs, and dark, creepy caves. Fake and misleading answers can pop out to fool you into thinking you don't require change and therefore allow you to justify remaining in a loop.

You see, in computer terms, your brain is hardware. Many of these mind patterns are software, and you have been using an outdated version! Time to upgrade your mind. You'll begin to enjoy the transformations and the new, more balanced being that is emerging.

When it comes down to it, as important as the other five aspects of optimal health are, until we realize that we are our patterns, we cannot successfully examine each aspect. We must recognize and preserve our good patterns, as well as analyze and change the patterns that no longer serve us.

Without the ability to change a bad pattern, we are in danger of staying in a state of imbalance. And for most, this state of imbalance can lead to harmful endings.

Mercury in Retrograde

It was late in the evening when the elderly, well-dressed gentleman quietly approached the front desk in the emergency department and asked to be seen as a patient. He was brought to a bed and chose to remain dressed in his tweed jacket and vest, rather than put on the ever-so-stylish and comfortable hospital gown.

We were busy, very busy. But I kept looking over at him as he comfortably read the newspaper, not appearing to be in any distress. He saw that it was very busy and was about to leave when I walked over to his bedside.

His complaint was a burning sensation when he urinated, with no explanation or obvious cause. With a negative history and physical exam, only the lab tests produced a clue. The urine test indicated evidence of an infection and possible trauma.

I don't know why—it was a gut instinct—but I ordered an X-ray of his abdomen and pelvis.

When the tech brought the films down for me to view, I saw three thermometers that he had inserted through his penis. Two were lodged in his urethra. The third was all the way in his bladder and had shattered! Needless to say, he was admitted for emergency surgery. He recovered well and was eventually discharged.

Two weeks later he was back with the same urinary complaints. He had repeated his maneuvers, and once again, more thermometers had been inserted! We, as the medical team, had done a great job treating his acute problem, but we had failed to treat the underlying pathological pattern of behavior.

Caring for people who show up at the hospital is always interesting, unique, and challenging. One would assume people who come with a problem want it fixed. So, when looking back on this case, I wondered why he would offer a chief complaint of "urinary burning" rather than "I shoved three thermometers up my schmiggie, and now I need help."

Of course, at the time I realized he had a psychiatric issue, but in "The Pit" on that particular evening, the physical problems had to take priority over the psychological. I arranged his admission to surgery and assumed a stay in the hospital would address all his issues.

Part of life is about learning lessons. It is said that if you learn the lesson, you move on; if you don't, the lessons become more painful. You also never know from whence the lesson or teacher appears.

In this case, I learned two great lessons from our gentleman with the "urinary burning".

Lesson 1: I had made the assumption that while he recovered in the hospital the initial cause of his issue would be addressed.

In medicine—and a few other things—I no longer *assume*.

I can assure you, the psychiatric issues were covered during his second admission.

Lesson 2: Any decision I have to make, I prioritize with one simple question: "Is this LIFE, LIMB, or SIGHT threatening?"

If the answer is yes, I make an immediate decision.

If no, I take my time to fully address the underlying aspects of the presenting condition.

Every once in a while in my personal life, someone might get annoyed when I don't make a decision as rapidly as they want. I've actually been accused of being "incapable of making decisions." I just sit back and quietly smile, reflecting on the life-and-death decisions that I do make.

The Cure

In medicine at the current time, with certain particular conditions such as cancerous states, we don't use the word *cure* much anymore. We instead offer various types of remission—even up to complete remission. But even that is complete only if the cancer doesn't return.

The herpes virus is usually not "cured." It, too, merely goes into remission until something wakes it from its hibernation.

Some medical professionals don't even consider that we "cure" strep throat with antibiotics. When you get it a second time, is it new or is it simply coming out of remission?

At this point we are only on the brink of changing outcomes with genetic engineering, and the future will be even more open to possibilities. We may actually have some cures!

But what if we think of some patterns of behavior in the same way? Meaning, if you have worked tirelessly to cure a bad pattern of behavior, but you can't—maybe you might want to shift the way you look at it: Mind Shift! Just try to put it in remission. Maybe one day it will go into complete remission!

The "cure" for life is truly putting *anything* causing pain and suffering—whether physical or mental—into remission.

KEEPING IT SIMPLE

From birth, we are constantly exhibiting patterns.

Recognize the patterns that don't serve you well—and change them.

Add new patterns that enhance and improve your life.

If you can't "cure" bad patterns, then at least attempt to put them into remission.

Chapter Seventeen

NUTRITION: A Twinkie a Day Keeps the Doctor in Business

*Men are not prisoners of fate, but
only prisoners of their own minds.*

—*Franklin D. Roosevelt*

As I arrived at the hospital for a morning shift, before I could even put my things down, the head nurse said, "Follow me. Now!"

When we came around the curtain, the patient in bed three was in the midst of a severe asthma attack, gasping for air—he was in *status asthmaticus*. The team was already working to help him: starting IV lines, putting him on oxygen, and prepping an intubation tray. I observed an extremely obese boy whose nine-year-old heart and lungs might not make it to the tenth.

He was taking his last few breaths.

His mother, sister, and brother were at his bedside with fearful, glassy expressions. They didn't fully comprehend the gravity of the situation, but intuitively each knew it wasn't good.

I encouraged the patient to enter a visualization mode with me. (I did this a lot with kids. It worked like a charm when they needed stitches.) The two of us focused on each other as he mimicked my breathing. With the right timing and appropriate medications, we were able to break the attack. The tide (of air, in this case) had turned; he was out of danger.

Almost as soon as he was able to breathe and speak, his mother looked at me and asked, "Is it okay to give him a bag of Cheetos? It's his favorite food."

Take a trip with me to the virtual laboratory, where we will put a one-celled organism in a petri dish. After the organism settles in and develops its own comfort zone, let's place a small amount of a toxic substance next to the cell.

What do you think the cell will do? You are correct; it will try to move away from the toxic substance in order to survive.

Now let's take the same little one-celled critter and place something near it that would be nutritional. Again, you are correct; the organism will move toward the nutrient.

The cell must always decide where to utilize its energy in survival (moving away from a toxin) or in growth and repair (moving toward a nutrient). Because it is just one cell, it can pretty much do only one at a time effectively.

Let us now take a giant leap into our own bodies, which are made up of millions and millions and millions of cells. Remember, in a metaphoric sense, we are made up of one-celled organisms all housed under the same roof.

Although the process is much more complex, it is helpful to understand that our cells are always trying to survive, grow, replicate, and perform their designated functions. When we ingest toxic substances (such as refined sugar, processed foods, or various chemicals) into our bodies, our cells will, in most circumstances, handle the substances effectively in order to survive—but at the price of growth and function.

Nutrition is clearly the most important aspect of optimal health. However, in my experience, it appears that some of you out there are more willing to take care of your businesses than your bodies and minds. If that is the case, here's a suggestion: Why not develop a mental model of your mind and body as a business plan?

Investment, growth and development, profit, sustainability, and environmental impact all seem to apply to our bodies as well as to our businesses. If you want a better OUTCOME, spend more time and energy on the IN-COME.

Many of the foods we are eating are getting worse. Most are produced with antibiotics, steroids, viral cocktails, various pesticides, and additives while also undergoing genetic modifications.

The foods we eat have contributed to an epidemic—correction—a *pandemic* of obesity. Consumers crave information about their food. Fully transparent labeling would provide the clarity necessary to make conscientious food choices. It's up to us to read and understand the intricacies and nuances of the labeling process as it exists. Consider educating yourself and participating in government legislation to provide more transparent and complete food labeling.

There is increasing corroboration that dietary habits influence the prevention, cause, and healing of many disease states. Overwhelming evidence now links nutrition to immune-system impairment, inflammation, obesity, heart disease, stroke, type 2 diabetes, and certain forms of cancer. (As research continues in the future, we can expect more links to even more maladies.)

In our modern world, it has become essential to consider special-needs diets such as gluten-free, lactose-free, low-sodium, ketogenic, diabetic, weight-reduction or weight-gain, and certainly, pre- and postoperative diets. Hippocrates said, "Let food be your medicine and medicine be your food" (although he said it in Greek).

As a Medical Guide, I offer my clients creative choices for nutrition based on Western and non-Western healing systems. As examples, traditional Asian medicine suggests eating cool foods when hot and hot foods when cool; Ayurvedic medicine emphasizes choosing certain foods (while avoiding others) based on body type. I encourage eating organic, eating more in tune with nature, and eating locally sourced and seasonal foods.

It's all about balance. Remember, Goldilocks ate the porridge that was "just right."

Carbs Are Too Complex

As I scan the literature daily, there are new and conflicting reports on just about everything we ingest: foods, supplements, minerals, vitamins, and chemicals. There are substances we apparently need to protect us from other substances we don't even know a lot about!

Nutrition advisories are ever-changing. Sure, my mother gave me cod liver oil, but she never offered me coenzyme Q_{10}. First, they told us we needed vitamin E, but then later, it became dangerous for us to take! We were asked to raise our vitamin D levels but later discovered it may not help in the prevention of bone fractures or improvement in bone density.

It is important to keep up with the literature, but I believe there are a few guidelines that can always be applied.

- First and foremost, rely on our old friend the 80/20 rule. Taking it slowly will help most of us change from the "Finish everything on your plate; others are starving" mentality to a newer concept of eating to be healthy. Figure out how good your eating habits are, and then shoot for 80 percent good eating habits and only 20 percent not so good. Over time, as you start feeling better and the shopping, cooking, and ordering in restaurants become easier, you may suddenly find you have arrived at a higher percentage.

- Don't ever "diet." Instead, adopt a nutrition plan. Ideas such as "Eat for your blood type" and "Eat for your Ayurvedic body type" are all parts of the puzzle. But we still don't know it all! Soon, your personal biome may dictate what is best for you. For now, your nutrition plan should be noninflammatory and include all the micro- and macronutrients that meet your personal needs.

- Look for healthy, organic, fresh food that makes you feel good after you eat it. Every good food is not necessarily agreeable to every *body*. Be discerning and scientific in your choices.

- If you find you have allergies or adverse reactions to specific foods, stop eating them. (Feel free to insert the old "Doctor, it hurts when I do this" joke.)

- Remember those cells I keep mentioning? Don't fool yourself; food may begin its journey as pizza, caviar, or a sandwich, but once your teeth and saliva kick into action, all the foods we eat make their way to those cells as proteins, fats, carbs, vitamins, and minerals. Those cells need—I said NEED (okay, I guess I didn't really *say* it, I wrote it)—proteins and complex carbohydrates and good, healthy fats. Diets and processed foods that eliminate any of those three may serve some purposes, but certainly *not* healthy purposes.

- Before eating, in order to combine spirituality and mindfulness with nutrition, create a moment to quiet yourself and give thanks in the form of gratitude. It doesn't have to be a religious blessing, but just a moment to reflect. Here's one version of my moment before a meal:

> *I give gratitude to all in nature that helped to provide this meal.*
>
> *I give gratitude to all those who produced the food and made it possible for me to bring it to my table.*
>
> *I give gratitude for my life and the ability to enjoy this meal.*
>
> *I wish all people could enjoy this same meal.*

Here's another thought: maybe consider another moment at the end of a meal for more gratitude—a postprandial prayer.

> *It doesn't matter if your glass is half empty or half full, just be grateful you have a glass.*
>
> —*author unknown*

Eating Techniques

- Eat slowly—make it a mindful meditation. Savor each bite. This will cause you to eat less and therefore consume fewer calories, making for better weight control. Careful, unhurried chewing also allows you the ability to recognize unexpected, inedible hard objects (shells, bones, or pebbles). Your teeth will thank you; your dentist will miss the revenue.

- Speak only when your mouth is empty of morsels that could be spit upon another's plate or clothing. (That's a fancy way to say, "Don't talk with your mouth full." Yes, you have heard this one before, but it's worth repeating.)

- Stop before you are stuffed.

Any intelligent fool can make things bigger and more complex... It takes a touch of genius—and a lot of courage—to move in the opposite direction.

—*Albert Einstein*

Food Fight

Various foods seem in constant battle for the right to be at the top of the pyramid (or the plate). Who can keep track? Experts' advice about diet and nutrition seems to be ever changing.

Take snacks (of course, I'm talking about healthy ones), for example. Some say snacking throughout the day is beneficial because it keeps you in a steady state and prevents overeating at mealtime. At the opposite end of the table are those who suggest periods of fasting! They recommend you avoid snacks, allowing your digestion and hormonal activity (such as insulin) to rest and reenergize rather than work continuously.

With so many conflicting opinions, the question remains: Whom do you believe and follow?

The answer is *yourself.*

A man's most valuable trait is a judicious sense of what not to believe.

—*Euripides*

Cornucopia

Find the right diet for *your* health, not someone else's. Try different diet recommendations and evaluate how you react: your energy, mood, productivity, bowel function, and need for products sold in the pharmacy's digestion aisle. Keep in mind that if you've abused your body with a lot of junk for most of your life, your system will take time to adjust.

It's a good idea to observe from the moment you ingest a particular food until approximately three days afterward. To establish a baseline, eat a meal with corn (or something else that doesn't digest) and record its transit time from your mouth to the first sighting in your toilet bowl. This will give you the relative time period during which you should evaluate the results of future dietary delights.

After you've established your process, go through all your diet choices, take notes, make good observations, and choose the foods and dietary habits that work best for you. Your results with any given diet may not be the same as your neighbor's.

However, one recommendation seems to be universal: the importance of breakfast.

Breakfast does exactly what its name says, "breaks the fast." Obviously, it begins our daily fueling. But it also has the ability to alter our metabolism. Starting our day with a breakfast low in carbs, and including protein and "good" fats, might boost our metabolism to a higher rate.

Don't get hooked into a culturally traditional pattern of eating behavior. You can have soup for breakfast and scrambled eggs for dinner. But whatever you do, don't skip meals.

The brain is a sugar junkie, meaning it uses mainly glucose to function. So, if you have any plans to use your brain during the day, make sure it is running on quality fuel and not fumes, in a tank that's neither running on empty nor flowing over into your reserve unnecessarily. You must police your own brain's cravings. Your performance, along with your waistline, will depend on it.

Bon Appétit

Forget the old adage "You are what you eat." That is only a partial story. "You are what you *absorb*" should be the mantra. Because of our poor diets and the endless food additives in processed foods, we are coating the inner lining of our intestines with sludge—hindering absorption.

You should not only trust your gut; you should also respect it! Obstacles to proper function of the gastrointestinal (GI) tract include poor dietary habits, repeated use of antibiotics, lack of exercise, insufficient rest, and chronic physical and emotional stress.

Even if we are consuming good whole foods, vitamins, and antioxidants, they may not be getting absorbed! The digestive tract is a huge biochemical factory that prepares food for digestion and absorption.

If you don't think your GI tract is critical to your overall well-being, think about the times you have had an upset stomach, nausea, vomiting, constipation, abdominal pain, or diarrhea. Not pretty. In fact, the next time you're in a pharmacy, take a walk through the aisle—or aisles—dedicated to digestion. It's overwhelming!

The gastrointestinal system (especially the large intestine, containing our personalized, individualized bacterial biome) also serves as the home of 70 to 80 percent of our immune system and host defenses. It is one of the prime defenses of the body against ingested toxins and other foreign invaders remaining in food. Without it, we would be at the mercy of many pathological creatures (e.g., *Clostridium botulinum*, which causes botulism).

Although Hippocrates believed that all disease began in the gut, Western medicine informed us that not every disease originated there. Other worldwide healing systems, however, have never ceased their focus on the gut in terms of diagnosis and treatment.

Recently, moving back toward Hippocrates's belief, current research is once again focusing on many non-gastrointestinal diseases—especially those with chronic inflammatory components, such as heart disease and stroke—indeed having their origins in the gut.

Let's Take a Left Turn and Go Off-Roadin'

I'm going to take you on one of the most treacherous, toxic, and *important* paths you will ever be on, yet it is only about thirty feet long.

It begins at the mouth.

Just like Ulysses was tied to the mast to avoid the call of the Sirens, you might find yourself needing restraint from your attraction to the inviting, pouty, full lips and the soft tongue.

But beware!

Hiding behind the lips and around the tongue are deadly structures known as teeth, capable of ripping flesh and crushing bone. And as if that weren't enough danger, because of the bacteria found in the mouth, a human bite can cause one of the worst infections known—that is, *if* you are lucky enough to get away from the grip!

For intended food, there is almost no escape, as saliva begins breaking down bitten-off, tasty morsels almost immediately. Then multiple, powerful muscles in the esophagus propel that crushed and shredded former food into the stomach, where it is bathed in gastric hydrochloric acid capable of destroying metal!

Leaving the stomach and entering the rugged terrain of the small intestine, what's left of the food is now exposed to alkaline bile juices that continue the breakdown process. Absorption into the blood and lymph streams begins. Eventually, food—or what's left of it that hasn't been absorbed—leaves the small intestine and enters the large intestine, a.k.a. the colon.

Here is an equally wild landscape. The food is exposed to a multitude of bacteria that complete its final breakdown and establish waste products to be evacuated (rather than remain in the body at harmful levels).

This metabolic process yields one of the most treacherous parts of our journey—an environment filled with toxic gases, such as methane and sulfur dioxide. Some of these same noxious gases are found in volcanoes.

(As a medical student, studying the intestinal tract, I learned two of my lifelong favorite medical terms: *putrescine* and *cadaverine*. These are products produced by bacterial breakdown of amino acids. You can imagine how foul-smelling they are just by their names—the smell present around rotting flesh.)

We are coming to the end of this trek. Let us take a moment of gratitude for all that has been accomplished in the metamorphosis of food into essential nutrients and waste.

And now let us take one last moment for the pièce de résistance. All hail the anal sphincter! This "exit ramp" of our off-road journey is a small group of muscles capable of magically recognizing and differentiating gas, liquids, and solids. It allows discriminatory and separate passage without even utilizing our usual senses of sight, touch, smell, etc. That's quite an accomplishment. Indeed, all hail.

So, we've finished our off-road adventure from the mouth to the anus, traveling only about thirty feet within the body. However, if you were to stretch out the internal mucosa of the small and large intestines, it would magnify to around half the square footage of a badminton court!

(Okay, I can barely picture that either, but I wanted to mention badminton because one of my brothers, a superb, award-winning athlete and personal trainer, was a badminton champion. And I also wanted to spell *badminton* multiple times.)

Let's Talk Tongue

I suppose while I am in a hailing mood, looking back, I really should have mentioned a few additional things about the amazingness of the tongue.

1. It not only helps move food out of the mouth and into the long digestive journey, but without it we wouldn't have clear speech and the ability to communicate in the way we do.

2. Okay, I should mention that it is a pretty sexy structure, but I'll leave that to your own imagery.

3. The tongue also has philosophical implications. There is a Chinese proverb, "The tongue is soft and remains; the teeth are hard and fall out," suggesting to us we should be softer in dealing with ourselves and others.

4. If we didn't have a tongue, how would we snag those little annoying food particles that get stuck between our teeth?

5. Traditional Asian medicine (TAM), as well as medicine from other cultures and healing systems, uses the tongue as an integral part of a medical examination. A TAM doctor carefully inspects many aspects of your tongue to determine the correct diagnosis and treatment. Conversely, we practitioners of Western medicine use an unappetizing, flat wooden stick to cover your tongue and move it down and away—ignoring the tongue and its secrets entirely. At the same time, we instruct you to say, "A A A A A HHHH," and potentially make you gag a little in the process. (In fact, I'm sure if I asked you right now to

say, "AAAAAHHHH," you would clench up in preparation to receive a wooden stick instead of purring, "aaaaaaahhhhhh," as though you were relaxed, meditative, and in a good state of mind.) I have often wondered why there is such a difference between Eastern and Western medicine in the level of respect for the tongue.

6. The tongue combined with saliva, according to the Taoists, is useful as a form of substitute toothbrush. They advise: run your tongue around each surface (upper-outer, upper-inner, lower-outer, lower-inner, and upper and lower grinding surfaces) nine times each, mixing with saliva. At the end, swish the saliva and swallow in three swallows.

All these functions should be enough for one small body part. But as they used to say on TV, "Wait, there's more," and it could be the tongue's most important function. Our taste buds, found on the anterior surface of the tongue, are sensory organs giving us the sensation of flavor and taste.

Some would disagree and say that it is not in truth "flavors," but rather the *qualities* of the ingredients that are being recognized—and recognizing these qualities helps us survive.

Sweet things communicate to us that they might be good for energy. A sour taste might indicate that something is no longer fresh and safe to eat (except for sour cream with fruit, of course). A bitter flavor might alert us to something toxic and therefore dangerous. A salty taste might be a warning the item is not healthy for consumption.

The flavor of umami, a recently recognized taste often described as "meaty," might suggest something benefiting the immune system. As we chew our way into the future, additional tastes may be discovered.

At one time or another, many of us have frustratedly expressed that the most difficult-to-remember, barely retrievable facts are stored at the "tip of the tongue." Perhaps scientists may uncover that memory is, indeed, a taste! (And I say that tongue-in-cheek.)

There is also what chefs call "mouth feel." Fats might suggest that a food is nutritious for the body, while the sensation of heat might help us avoid a burn to the mouth or esophagus.

The tongue is amazing, is it not? And, at some point in your life, you may even run into someone with extraordinarily acrobatic tongue skills. They may be able to curl it, fold it, or tie a knot in a cherry stem with it.

No One Likes to Lose

Words matter.

Most overweight to morbidly obese people always—I say, *always*—try to lose weight. Logically. But in my mind, that means the deck is already stacked. You will lose to the house. (Sorry, I flashed back to a casino table for a moment. Okay, I'm back.)

No one likes to lose!

We don't want to lose a set of keys, a wallet, a phone, a favorite jacket, our other glasses, a pet, or a loved one.

I repeat: *No one likes to lose!*

So, I suggest, don't *lose* weight; *gain* health with every pound.

KEEPING IT SIMPLE

This was a complicated chapter, so let me digest it for you:

We eat every day; we might as well make it a healthy practice.

As Michael Pollan advises in *In Defense of Food*:

1. Eat real food, not chemicals.

2. Eat less food.

3. Eat mainly plant-based food.

And I would like to add:

4. Although it's technically not food, drink water.

 To stay hydrated and discover more insights on water consumption, visit **GlennWollman.com/resources** and check out Guidepost 14—Watch the Road Signs: Water Hazard.

All you need is love. But a little chocolate now and then doesn't hurt.

—Charles Schulz

Chapter Eighteen

PHYSICAL ACTIVITY: "Give Me Four More!"

Working the night shift in Beverly Hills was fun because the police would hang out with us during quiet times. It was always great telling stories around the old otoscope light (which we used to simulate a campfire).

One officer wanted some medical advice, and I was happy to help. He complained of intermittent headaches, neck aches, and lower-extremity joint pains. He had already received an extensive medical workup and no significant pathology had been found. Frankly, at this point, he wanted to make sure it wasn't psychosomatic and that the doctors hadn't missed something ominous.

After taking a thorough history and reviewing all the studies he had already received, I was able to deduce that his symptoms would manifest following his exercise regimen: running five miles every morning and five miles every evening. (He was a seasoned officer who wanted to set an example for the younger rookies.)

Like all habitual runners, he loved it and couldn't live without it (you know... the endorphin high). He didn't want to stop, but as an experiment, he begrudgingly agreed to cease and desist for two weeks.

Okay, as I'm sure you already guessed, his symptoms all disappeared. He was feeling great. He was thrilled.

At the end of the successful two-week experiment, he had a decision to make. He had been enjoying a pain-free life for the first time in many years.

He lasted a week and then started running again. All of his symptoms immediately returned.

At least he was relieved to know it wasn't all in his head. Or was it? It was a pattern of behavior he was unwilling to change. Continuing to choose running as his form of physical activity despite its accompanying issues was harmful, even under the guise of health.

It is more and more evident that we must exercise—every day. The frequency, duration, and intensity are still part of the question. Exercise is extremely important, but not when it is causing more damage. One thing is clear: especially as we get older, the mantra "No pain, no gain" should be replaced by "No pain, NO PAIN!"

In fact, while we're replacing accepted terminology, I'd prefer we focus less on the word *exercise* and more on the all-encompassing and much less intimidating concept of *physical activity*. I have no doubt that physical activity is the most important aspect of optimal health.

Making a small change from an inactive lifestyle to one that includes periodic but regular movement and activity can help prevent disease and premature death, and improves quality of life. If we reconsider inactivity as a *disease* with many consequences (including a higher incidence of mortality), then we can certainly proclaim activity as the cure.

Sitting Moves You

As research has shown, prolonged sitting (for periods longer than twenty minutes) is a rapid way to move closer to a coffin. So, for all of you stuck in front of a computer all day long, consider this simple, effective countermeasure:

Stand up every twenty minutes and do your ABCs:

Align: Check your posture. Balance equally on both feet and attempt to stand one inch taller than your slouching stance.

Breathe: Perhaps utilize the Wollman Meta4 Square Breath I'll discuss later in Chapter 20. It only takes about sixty-four seconds. (Come on. There's no excuse for not having sixty-four seconds to devote to your physical activity.)

Calm: Clear your mind of all thoughts and honor the moment. Don't worry, all your thoughts will still be there when you sit again. This moment of calm may even help solve a problem or offer an insight into your current work.

Many of today's desks are designed for both sitting and standing. However, this short respite of light activity (as well as the occasional stretch or walk to the bathroom) is still a good idea for physically getting away from your desk as well as mentally regrouping.

Moving On

Physical activity should be personal, based on lifestyle and needs, but don't limit yourself to only one form of exercise. The really good news is that there are so many great choices to make physical activity fun. There are options for indoor, outdoor, seasonal, solitary, and group programs: Pilates, yoga, martial arts, swimming, surfing, snowboarding, kayaking, hiking, basketball, volleyball, tennis, badminton (help... I can't stop writing that), and dancing, just to name a few.

For me, the gym is an excellent place to get my activity: mental, physical, and also social. But tread carefully. The gym is also a place where one can get hurt—and, believe me, I speak from multiple experiences.

(Marital disclaimer: My wife fervently believes that everyone should head directly to a Pilates studio. Under the guidance of an expert instructor like my wife, movements are designed for each individual to be constructive rather than potentially destructive. But I'll let her write her own book!)

To Gym or Not to Gym

First, you must make the decision that working out with weights, equipment, and machines in an indoor setting with many other people is your preference. Joining a gym certainly serves many purposes, not the least of which is avoiding the expensive purchase of an apparatus for your home (which, in most cases, eventually becomes a very large, irregularly shaped clothes hanger).

But let's be fair, there are advantages and disadvantages to the gym.

Advantages:

- Usually, good, modern equipment is available and always being upgraded.

- A social aspect can motivate you to work out with others like yourself.

- There may be a sauna or steam room.

- There may be a Jacuzzi or pool.

- There is usually an assortment of classes. Stretching, yoga, Pilates, or aerobic kickboxing might be available.

- Experts may be available to advise you on proper form and routine.

- Last but not least: you will be seen next to people who are lesser physical specimens than you!

Disadvantages:

- Inconvenience: you will have to travel from your home.

- You may prefer movement outside in the fresh air, as opposed to exercising indoors.

- Gyms can be expensive.

- Last, but again, not least: you will be seen next to people who are in much better shape than you!

Gym Pickings: Choosing Your Gym

- Find a facility that is located either close to your home or near your place of work, depending on whether you plan to go when you are not working or would prefer to go during your lunch break. If your gym is too far away and not convenient, you will tend not to go. It's human nature.

- Make sure there is adequate parking with easy access. Too many times I have driven to the gym when I was only partly in the mood to work out. When I found no parking, it conveniently became *"not my fault"* that I had to turn around and go home. (Can I blame human nature again?)

- Check out your potential gym at the specific time of day you will usually be there. If it's too crowded at that time, you might have to "wait for the weight." This lag time can throw you off your routine and discourage you from returning regularly.

Preworkout

It should go without saying, but make sure you have had plenty of rest. Exercising while exhausted is a recipe for injury.

At least two or three hours before your workout, have a light meal that consists of good protein balanced with healthy fats and complex carbohydrates. You need the protein to build those muscles you'll be working hard to attain, and you need the fats and carbs for fuel so you don't "bonk" during the workout.

If you have a craving for sweets or caffeine, have them only in small amounts before the workout. I don't recommend them as a habit, but I will admit it is less harmful to have them at this time rather than as a midnight snack.

At the beginning of my workout at the gym, I spend about fifteen to twenty minutes in moving meditation (Qigong). I do this in a quiet place to de-stress, focus my *attention* on where I am, and stop thinking about other things. Doing an exercise while thinking about other things is a very good formula for getting hurt.

I also assert my *intention* during this meditation: "I intend to create harmony of body, mind, and spirit for the purpose of achieving optimal health through my practice."

To accomplish that intention, it is critical to UNPLUG! No texting, emailing, or checking Instagram. Leave the outside world behind and focus on yourself.

The Workout

After about sixty to ninety minutes, certain hormones in the body kick in to defeat the purpose of weight training. So, keep to your routine but keep that routine limited to only ninety minutes *at the most* for each workout.

High-intensity interval training (HIIT) was originally designed for athletes and other physical competitors such as bodybuilders. But for the rest of us, it is a very efficient way to accomplish a full workout in less time. Do your research (perhaps investigate Tabata, a type of HIIT) and seek professional advice before embarking.

Especially during HIIT, don't focus so intently on getting in a certain number of reps during a certain time frame that you forfeit proper form and technique (another formula for injury).

Don't forget to breathe and hydrate! Breathe during and between sets (groups of repetitions of exercises), and hydrate between sets.

Make all your exercises and movements a diagnostic procedure. Consider it "diagnostics with benefits." If all is well, then continue with the movement or sport and enjoy the benefits.

But at any time, if anything hurts, *stop immediately*. Pain is an indicator that something is not right. Honor it. Otherwise, an injury may keep you out of the gym for an extended period of time—possibly even requiring therapy or surgical procedures to resolve.

There are many different types of pain. With time, you might be able to discern the difference between nerve, muscle, tendon, or ligament pain. For the most part, it is good to stop immediately when you feel *any* type of pain.

Okay, this next tip is really important and might be extremely helpful as a clue to relay to an orthopedic surgeon (should you require one). At the first onset of pain, etch in your memory whether you heard any sound or sounds. Don't forget them. Perhaps write them down, on the off chance that you need clarity when you report them later.

Depending on the type and intensity of the injury, there are two sounds you may hear. The first is the more important: a popping or clicking. This might be indicative of ligament or tendon involvement.

The second sound you may hear is you, screaming an expletive as you realize you just messed up.

After you've acknowledged any sounds accompanying your injury, look at the painful area. Is there any bleeding, any swelling, or—perish the thought—something sticking out through your skin?

If no, feel the area to see if it hurts to the touch. If the area hurts to the touch, it is a good idea to stop that exercise and deal with the issue—based on the amount of pain and limitation of motion.

If it doesn't hurt to the touch, check for pain on passive range of motion—meaning you move the joint with your hand. If it doesn't hurt on passive motion, then check it out with active motion—using the muscles in that area to move the joint. Finally, test it by doing the exercise you were working on when the pain began, but with very light weight. Sometimes it will be better, but if it still hurts, stop and let it rest! Move on to a different muscle group or seek immediate professional attention.

Remember I suggested earlier that you get an anatomy reference book? Well, learning the muscles you'll be exercising will help you focus on using correct form during your workout. You will hopefully remember about origin, insertion, and action. Maybe you'll even have some familiarity with nerve supply, in case of an injury.

And, speaking of injuries, knowing more of the human anatomy may help you, while you are practicing being your own health-care provider, to make a good potential diagnosis and might guide you on the path to prevent further injury.

More Is Sometimes Too Much

We of course know that too little exercise is unhealthy, but science is proving that *overdoing* exercise is also harmful to the heart and other structures. Don't forget Goldilocks. Keep your exercise regimen juuuuuuust right.

In fact, although contrary to established wisdom for muscle enlargement (and not meant for supreme athletes and professionals), this may be the most important of all my "gym tips": if you are struggling to complete the last one or two repetitions in your predetermined set, such that you are giving up form and technique, DON'T COMPLETE THE SET. If you have reached exhaustion, the last two reps are prime time for disaster.

Based on how many times I have treated athletic injuries, I feel obligated to remind you, an injury can be costly in terms of time, money, discomfort, and fun.

So, while you thought my gym tip was to simply forgo the last one or two reps to avoid injury, that was merely the beginning. My *real* advice is to develop a new pattern of behavior. Unless you integrate this self-awareness and discipline ahead of time—prep, practice, and plan it—you will probably make the wrong decision in the moment.

Remember: You are not attempting to win a gold medal! The real win is improving yourself and doing better today than you did yesterday.

KEEPING IT SIMPLE

- Have pieces of equipment strategically placed all around your home. This will enable you to stay active even while your attention cannot be devoted fully to exercise. A level of mindlessness for simpler moves can be acceptable, so that they can be performed while on the phone, sitting at the computer, etc. For example, I use the Pilates Magic Circle while watching television.

- Frequency:

  - Include 150 minutes per week of aerobic, mind/body activity, balance work, and stretching.

  - Incorporate an additional 40 to 60 minutes per week of resistance or weight training.

- Intensity:

  - At the end of an exercise, you should endeavor to be winded enough so as not to be able to sing "Row, Row, Row Your Boat" for about a minute.

- The One-Set Routine:

Do this—very, very, very slowly—every day you are unable to do a regular workout.

  - Take one deep breath. As you let it out—very slowly but continuously—tighten every muscle in your body in a sequence from head to toe or from toe to head. Hold all the muscles tight until you finish the exhale. (This is one that can be done almost anywhere.) Then do:

  - One pushup

  - One situp (modified to protect your back)

  - One plank

  - One calf raise (one done with each calf, Smarty-Pants)

- ○ One knee bend (yes, with both knees, Double Smarty-Pants)

- ○ One chinup (if you have access to a chinup bar. Oh, and for this you can use only one chin, unless you have a double chin. Okay, so now *I'm* Dr. Smarty-Pants.)

The theory? Doing one is better than doing none. And, once you're busy doing one, you might be inspired to do two!

Chapter Nineteen

SLEEP MANAGEMENT:
Vitamin Zzzzzzz

After a busy night shift, the emergency department physician turned over all his cases to the oncoming doctor and packed his gear to go home. On the two-lane, country highway, he fell asleep at the wheel and crashed into a parked car.

A few days later, another physician was on her way to work after a poor night of angst-filled sleep and fell asleep at the wheel, crashing into a tree. Even though we were trained not to sleep, even we doctors need it.

While we still don't know everything about sleep, we're continually learning how poor sleep patterns can result in long-term pathology manifested in diseases or disorders. If you are not really sure sleep is important, here's a good test. Perform a few mental and physical tests (such as math or coordination movements) and mark down the results. Then, avoid sleep for as many days as you can and repeat the tests, comparing results.

You may be so sleep-deprived that you cannot adequately take the tests or objectively interpret the results. So, perhaps do all this with someone who is willing to watch over you.

Your friend may want to video this experiment so that you can observe the results when you're more rested. And who knows? It might even be funnier than a cat video.

And by the way: *Don't actually try that experiment!* An extreme lack of sleep would obviously be unsafe, but the thought of it should make my point.

We obsess over cholesterol levels and other chemical markers but ignore this very critical component of our balance. So, I consider sleep to be the most important aspect of optimal health because it is so integral to our daily ability to address the other aspects.

We have become a sleep-sick society with the number of people with sleep disorders rising to epidemic proportions. We certainly don't want our surgeons, air traffic controllers, or school bus drivers afflicted.

There is no argument that we need sleep. But how much? The traditional consensus is we need around seven and a half to eight hours of sleep per night. Many of us have friends who claim they don't need that much. They are wrong—they just may not know it yet.

Sleep is the primary time the brain eliminates certain types of waste products and toxins. Who wants a dirty mind?

You can determine the amount of sleep you require based on your next day's performance: the yawn count, number of head nods, body jerks in your chair, and chin crashes on your desk.

But regardless of the *quantity* of sleep one prefers, we can all agree that achieving high-quality sleep is most beneficial.

In Search of a Good Night's Sleep

Experts have provided a plethora of information on the value of sleep and methods to improve sleep (including sleep diaries). I encourage you to take advantage of their in-depth research. However, here are some of my selected sleep strategies:

- **Honor sleep**! Sleep is as valid to your life experience as waking activities are.

- Cut down on stimulants, nicotine, and alcohol.

- Exercise regularly but not right before sleep time.

- Unwind early in the evening.

- Develop a sleep ritual.

- Create a restful place to sleep.

- Decrease light and brightness.

- Give yourself "permission" to go to bed.

- Sleep on a comfortable, supportive mattress and foundation. Love your bed.

- Use the bed for sleep and sexual activity only. Try to avoid other activities in bed unless they help you fall asleep.

How to Wake Up

Everyone focuses on the "sleep" part of sleep, but I'd like to highlight another important aspect: waking up!

Follow my path, yet feel free to be creative with the template:

- At the moment you awaken as your consciousness is returning, continue to keep your eyes closed and slowly turn over onto your back.

- Lie perfectly still and welcome yourself back to the universe.

- With your eyes still closed, continue to lie perfectly still—without any movement. Begin a virtual body scan. I usually start at my toes and work my way up to my head. If you notice anything new or out of the ordinary (pain or discomfort), make a mental note and move on to the next step.

- Test all your joints and muscles, beginning with your toes. With very minimal movement, slowly move your toes in all directions: flex, extend, spread apart, and squeeze together. Progress upward to your ankles, again moving them in many directions. Move on to your knees and then to your hips. Continuing with minimal movement, flex and extend with both outward and inward rotations. Look for pain or discomfort. If you feel no pain, continue. If there is any discomfort, acknowledge it and keep mental notes. Move to your pelvis and then up your spine all the way to your neck, continuing with small movements in all directions. Move down your arms from your shoulders to your elbows, wrists, and fingers. Finally, turn your attention to your face. Make lots of expressions involving your eyes, lips, tongue, and so on.

- At this point you have welcomed yourself back to awareness by doing two virtual body scans: one without movement followed by one with minimal movements.

- If you found no discomfort or pain, spectacular! If you notice discomfort in one or more places, lie there for a while to see if a little more movement will improve or aggravate the issue. (These areas will need to be addressed once you get out of bed.)

- Once you have done your body check, it's time to go to a mind check. Are you thinking clearly, awakening from sleep well? Or are you groggy and possibly in need of more sleep?

- Keeping your eyes closed, begin to set a few goals for the day or form some affirmations. For example: "Today I am going to make people smile and laugh." "Today I am going to be helpful to friends and strangers." "Today I will appreciate things." One of the most deeply influential elements of successfully waking up is having meaning in life and a reason to get up and do things.

- Mentally note a few things you are grateful for and give thanks and appreciation for them.

- Finally, when all this is done (and, by the way, once you get good at it, it should take only a minute or two), open your eyes for the first time and let the light from within you intermingle and join with the light from the Universe.

Body? Check!
Mind? Check!
Spirit? Check!
This process will be the beginning of a great day.

Get out of bed slowly and in stages, being aware of the areas of discomfort you acknowledged during your body scan. Are those pains gone, or are they still there? If they're still there, check out the area more thoroughly with visual observation followed by palpation (touching). Perhaps you should consider having a particularly painful area evaluated by a professional.

As your day unfolds, use your mind to check in periodically with your body and spirit. Reevaluate the current condition of any physical discomfort and confirm that you have been doing whatever it was you chose as your theme for the day.

Have a spectacular day!

Before you go to sleep, evaluate whether or not you met your goals and held on to your gratitude throughout the day. Then have a good night's sleep!

KEEPING IT SIMPLE

Sleep affects metabolism, hormones, mood, the immune system, digestion... actually every system in your body.

Get the right amount of good sleep. Scientists recommend around eight hours of sleep every night. I recommend whatever amount proves best for you.

Too little and too much sleep can both cause harm.

Wake up well.

This chapter may have seemed a little short compared to the others, but that's my way of encouraging you to quit futzing around reading and *go to sleep*!

Chapter Twenty

STRESS MANAGEMENT: "I Think; Therefore, I'm Stressed"

I get up every morning determined to both change the world and have one hell of a good time. Sometimes this makes planning my day difficult.

—*E. B. White*

When people hear that I worked in an emergency department, they always respond with "I couldn't handle the stress!" The truth is I never consciously realized the stress, although after I stopped working, all the stress became apparent. It was exciting in the ED because we never knew who was coming in, with what, and when they would arrive.

How could I possibly conceive that the next patient would haunt me for the rest of my life?

Consider this last statement a warning! Skip to the end of this story if reading what haunted me may haunt you.

It was in the early afternoon on a weekday when the paramedic radio went off. I got my first clue that something was different, because while the paramedics usually sound cool and organized, this one had a very sad quality to her voice. They were bringing in a four-month-old baby girl in full cardiac and respiratory arrest. Our team geared up both physically and emotionally, because babies in distress trigger a protective, primitive response even in the most seasoned health-care providers.

My second clue was upon arrival. The paramedic was carrying the baby in her arms—not on a backboard. It was a "scoop-and-run," so we had to move quickly.

I immediately followed the ABCs of CPR, going right to the airway and doing an intubation so we could give the baby girl much-needed oxygen. While continuing CPR, the nursing team was able to start an IV with steady hands and great skill. (Imagine placing a small needle into a vein the size of a thread, while riding in a rickety stagecoach on a bumpy country road.)

Nobody knew what had happened to the baby. The seventeen-year-old father/boyfriend, who was babysitting his daughter while the fourteen-year-old mother/girlfriend was out shopping, didn't give us any helpful information.

As I undressed the baby and began my initial trauma survey, searching for clues that might suggest a cause and therefore a treatment, it became all too clear.

To this day, the vision of the father's boot print embossed on the tiny girl's torso from her pelvis to her chest is also embossed in my mind. The baby had been crying inconsolably, and the young parent had no coping skills or knowledge of how to comfort his baby daughter. The stress just pushed him over the edge.

S tress can cause inappropriate reactions, sometimes carrying the danger of irreversible consequences. Worse yet, many times the damage caused is subtle and not always obvious. Considering this potentially insidious harm, is it any wonder I list stress management as the most important aspect of optimal health?

Stress involves hormones and neurotransmitters. The adrenal glands, for example, produce epinephrine (adrenaline) when you are angry, or in fear, or stressed, or running from an oncoming bus, or just excited on a giant roller coaster. The glands make no distinction of circumstance. Think about that—no distinction between an argument with your boss in your air-conditioned office or facing a robber at gunpoint.

Adrenaline and other hormones (such as cortisol) may be briefly beneficial, but prolonged production and excessive exposure can cause cellular harm. It's one of the few imbalances in our lives that has the potential to be dangerous not only to ourselves but also to *those around us.*

Intermittent explosive disorder (for example, road rage) precipitates abnormal behavior resulting in injury to ourselves and others through accidents. Adding "insult to injury," those accidents then may result in expensive costs, property damage, liability, and medical bills.

It is well accepted from many scientific studies that prolonged stress can raise our potential to have heart attacks and strokes by increasing risk factors.

We must address stress before it addresses us. Meditation, mindfulness, stress reduction techniques, and professional help are great approaches. There are myriad techniques! I suggest you possess a number of them that work for you. Here's one you might like:

The Wollman Meta4 Square Breath

I devised this technique based, of course, on all the work that people throughout the ages have done on "the breath." I have used it myself over and over in the emergency department during some of the worst crises. For example...

Never mind, let's not get sidetracked away from the technique.

Practice this technique consistently *before* you are in a stressful situation. Repetitive practice develops neural pathways that can be called upon during high-stress moments—preventively. When stressed, just beginning the Wollman Meta4 Square Breath can trigger the newly created neural pathways and reduce stress with more immediacy.

Here's the big picture. (Okay, it's actually a medium picture.)

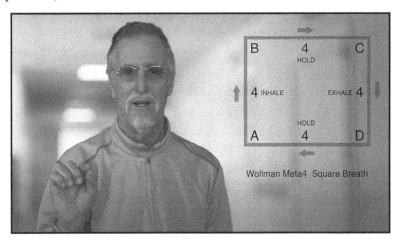

View a full video overview of the Wollman Meta4 Square Breath at **GlennWollman.com/meta4**

- Imagine a square
- Begin in the bottom-left corner (A) of the square. Breathe in through your nose along the left line

of the square going upward (A–B) and make the inhale last—slowly and comfortably—for four seconds.

- Along the top line (B–C) of the square, hold the inhaled breath comfortably for four seconds.

- On the right line, from top to bottom (C–D), exhale through your mouth for four comfortable seconds.

- And finally, on the bottom line from right to left (D–A), hold the exhale by not breathing until you arrive at the lower-left corner (A) again in four seconds.

- Start over again with the inhale, and repeat the entire process four times.

Four parts, four seconds each part, four times around the square, repeated four times a day. Breathing **four square!**

Many forms of meditation support other breathing techniques. However, my method may be incorporated into other breathing patterns to begin the de-stress/relaxation process.

Advanced Details:

Instead of expanding your chest when you breathe in, expand your abdomen by using your diaphragm. When you exhale, your tummy should flatten. This technique (diaphragmatic breathing) is used by meditators, martial artists, singers, and musicians. It may take a little while to perfect, but I advise that you pursue it, as it is good to learn and will help in other areas. For example, it really comes in handy if you ever have chest wall pain or broken ribs, and you really feel the need to take a deep breath, but it hurts too much to expand your chest.

By the way, the four seconds is just to get you started. As you get better at this process, you may naturally desire each segment to last longer than four *seconds*. Follow your instincts. But even if the timing lengthens as you advance, always keep it as a count of four.

The last "four"—holding the exhale (D–A)—is probably the most difficult of all the sides of the square. Here is a tip: in order to extend holding the exhaled breath a bit longer, swallow some saliva or just dry swallow. This will give you a little more time.

Missing the Metaphor? Rounding the Square

Okay, I believe you understand the *4* in the name of my technique. "But where's the Metaphor?" you might ask.

This breathing exercise is a metaphor for the life cycle. To illustrate, join me on this trek around the square:

Following a brief glide (albeit from the mother's point of view not necessarily brief or a glide) from the uterus, through the vaginal canal, and out into civilization, the first thing a fetus does is announce its citizenship in the species. It takes a breath in: Point A. Inhale, inspire! And from the point of view of one who has delivered many fetuses, it *is* inspirational.

System dependence on Mom closes down and shuts off. The umbilical cord is severed. All the precious cells I have mentioned begin to rely on a new individual for their existence—suddenly preparing for a lifetime of growth, development, maintenance, decline, and death.

Completing the metaphor, just as the first thing the fetus does is inhale, the last thing an individual does when he or she leaves this planet is *exhale* (Point C). So, traveling the circle of life along the Meta4 Square serves as its own metaphor for life.

Each time you proceed through one Wollman Meta4 Square Breath, it is as though you are going through a lifetime— you are reborn; you die. Hindus believe that upon each rebirth, we become more enlightened. Through each Meta4 Square Breath, we strive to also become more enlightened by consciously considering its metaphor.

Neuroscientists studying accomplished meditators note that elongated exhalation improves the chances of reaching a meditative state. Each time after the first round, you should focus deeper and deeper on life. Look at each time 'round the square as a metaphorical rebirth. You should become better with each round. It is a meditative opportunity to make changes.

KEEPING IT SIMPLE

Recognize the triggers that cause stress.

Recognize the symptoms induced by stress.

Have a practiced routine to address the stress (e.g., Meta4 Square Breath or meditation).

If none of these work, see a professional.

Chapter Twenty-One

SPIRITUALITY: "If You Have Nothing to Be Grateful for, Check Your Pulse"

*Mind is reality. With one thought
you can be in heaven, with another, in hell.*

—Buddha

When the police come into the ED along with Child Protective Services, I usually expect an unhappy situation.

A family of multiple siblings, ranging from approximately two to eleven years old, was brought in. The clothing they wore suggested they were an extremely traditional, religious family. (Some of the limited information provided by the police and Child Protective Services helped confirm this initial observation.)

I was hoping it was food poisoning or an infection, such as ringworm or lice. Yet none of the children appeared to have obvious physical trauma or be in any acute distress—aside from it being late at night in an emergency department with police and CPS in attendance.

Whatever I expected, I was not prepared for this.

We learned that the parents had been molesting the older children for years. Now, as they began to molest the younger ones, they were forcing the older children to be a part of it.

The two oldest children, not yet even teenagers, had contacted the police.

The spirituality of the two older children—rather than the religion of the parents—will hopefully save and teach the younger siblings.

What I consider spirituality should not be confused with religion (although the two can intertwine). Spirituality, however, doesn't exist because of clothing, rituals, or customs. It exists within the heart-mind and is a guiding light to help us live within ourselves and be in harmony with others and our surroundings.

Early in my medical education, midway through, I studied traditional Asian medicine and the five elements: wood, fire, earth, metal, and water. I always wondered about the validity of air as an element. It was explained to me that air was in everything! In much the same way, spirit is like air. It is intangible, and we can't grasp it. Yet it touches everything, and we can see its effects.

Spirituality is profoundly personal. It's about being centered and having a connection to the bigger picture—the Universe and all living things. Without it, we are an illusion and don't recognize it. That is why spirituality is the most important aspect of optimal health—the aspect holding the key to making deep connections to all the others.

And who could argue this?

Spiritual Paradox

Humanity owes a great deal to all those throughout history who chose to be renunciates and ascetics. No matter what their religion or philosophy, the choice was to go deeply into the Inner Universe to find the path to enlightenment.

Externally, it appears that the paths may be different, but they all seem to have some commonality: each talks about profound love and compassion for all beings.

This path does not come without sacrifice. To learn these important lessons, the devoted are usually unable to experience the individual love of another person. Instead, their love is for all humankind and their Creator/God/Deities. They generally experience very little human touch, except during ceremonies and for the purpose of blessings, yet they have touched the world!

It's Cawma

Our experience with the spiritual can come in many forms.

Every year on my birthday, like clockwork, the plum tree in my backyard gives fruit as though it were my birthday present from nature. Unfortunately, as nature giveth, it also taketh away. Each year, the squirrels and birds increasingly eat the plums before I have a chance to collect them. I am always willing to share, but they are insatiable!

Over time, I tried to figure out a way to thwart their theft so I could have plums on my birthday. I tried a fake owl statue and hung waving streamers of silver foil, all to no avail.

Eventually, I decided to try netting surrounding the tree, draped all the way from the top so the birds couldn't get to the fruit and tied tightly at the bottom so the squirrels couldn't climb to swipe the fruit either. It seemed to be working. Daily, I observed the plums—and my desire for them—ripen, while just as importantly, I saw no evidence of decimated fruit.

Most mornings, I am awakened by the cawing of crows outside my window. But on the morning before one birthday, the sound was not normal. In fact, the sound was so different, I wasn't even sure it was a crow!

When I went out to the backyard to investigate, I found that a solitary crow had somehow entered the netting and was stuck inside. He was cawing in obvious distress and confusion. Adding to the caw-cophony were about thirty additional crows circling above—the trapped crow's peeps—noisily squawking in solidarity! As I decided to mount a rescue attempt, their angst heightened, forcing me to consider the potential of an aerial attack.

The panic-induced screaming from within the netting increased, as did the sympathetic screeching from above. It was getting crazy. I had to act quickly to release the ensnared crow. But I couldn't get the knots of the netting untied!

It seemed the only way to get in would be to tear the netting. I was hesitant, realizing my plums would then be completely accessible until new netting could be purchased and applied. But it had to be done. I ripped it apart.

I tried to reach inside to get the winged thief out, but it would flap to the other side of the tree, away from me. I decided to try to round it up, gently using a stick to direct it closer to me. Eventually, my strategy worked, and the crow came close enough that I could grab it with my hands and pull it out of the netting.

The backyard fell silent. I sat, holding it gently in my hands for a moment to convey that I intended it no harm and that it wasn't going to get hurt. When I felt the bird relax, I released it into the air, where it joined all the other crows as they circled around and flew away.

Suddenly, the freed crow came back and stood by me. We shared a few quiet moments, and then it left.

At that point, it was all over...

Except for the fact that now, everywhere I go, a crow appears.

Even in places that don't make sense—places you wouldn't expect to see a crow, like at the beach—one is always there and usually walks alongside me. I resist the idea that it's anything more than coincidence, but my wife takes great pleasure in pointing out, "There's your crow!"

Fast-forward to about a year—and many crow instances—later. I was at the gym in a quiet little outdoor courtyard space where I practice Qigong and meditation before lifting weights or doing cardio. I relish the quiet peace of this space.

Unexpectedly, my cherished silence was interrupted by a guy screaming into his cell phone. Apparently, he was talking to his sister about their father's irresponsible housekeeper. How do I know these intimate details? Because he was yelling so loudly into the phone, the woman on the other end of the call was forced to shout over him. The sheer volume left me unable to escape hearing both ends of the conversation.

I thought it would stop in a second, but it went on and on and on and on and...

I started to get frustrated, but I said to myself, "This is an opportunity to practice my deeper meditation!" I was able to overcome the challenge of the noise for a momentary meditation, then I would pop out of it; a little more meditation, and then I would come out again. This wasn't working.

I was about to give up, when somewhere in my consciousness I became aware of a familiar cawing from above.

Suddenly, the guy on the phone screamed at the top of his lungs, "OH, NO!! I'm getting bombarded by a crow! It's POOPING on me!" With that, he ran back into the building.

It was quiet again, and I returned to my meditation with a wry smile on my face in appreciation of my ever-present crow.

So, Bird Poop Is Spiritual?

Now, you may be thinking that reaction doesn't sound incredibly spiritual on my part. But in my defense—not that I need one—I certainly experienced gratitude for the crow, while also feeling empathy for the loud, crow-poop-target guy. The moment did beautifully illustrate our interconnectedness with both nature and each other, key parts of spirituality.

Let's face it, even humor is a manifestation of spirituality.

Since we're on the subject, in what other ways is spirituality manifested? For me it is gratitude, compassion, happiness, character, forgiveness, empathy, morals, ethics, trust, creativity, education, courage, equanimity, and humor. (Please feel free to fill in other attributes that resonate with you.) But keep in mind, this list is not just an inventory of words. Each word is a practice unto itself. A constant practice.

For instance, it's not enough to feel gratitude only when your dreaded MRI or lab test is declared normal. Nay, nay, nay, my fellow wayfarers. You must make gratitude (and humor and empathy, et al.) an integral part of your daily spiritual life.

On the whole, spirituality is a guide for how to live your best life and die your best death.

My time in the emergency department provided me with opportunities to be present as patients approached death. Those with an established spiritual practice transitioned gracefully away from life. Those who had no such practice had anything but a smooth death. I watched many people hurriedly try to develop a spiritual practice in their final moments. Occasionally, it worked, but for the most part, it didn't.

My experience should serve as a reminder to begin a daily spiritual practice now. There's only so much sand in the hourglass.

Mind Travel

I hope I've encouraged you to step back into the bookstore and comb the appropriate shelves for expert, in-depth instruction and advice regarding nutrition, physical activity, and sleep and stress management. I also encourage you to find additional spiritual guidance and support. Perhaps it may come in the form of a book, or perhaps it may come as a teacher or guru.

As usual, though, I do have a few tips that I've utilized. But before I share my specific meditations, let me briefly return to the topic of breathing—one of the most basic yet most important tools in learning how to meditate.

When the body initially forms, the most primitive portion of the brain—the brain stem—begins to develop. Through the brain stem, we develop the processes for some of our basic vital life patterns: heartbeat (rate and rhythm), breathing, temperature control, and sleep-wake cycles, to name a few. In the same way we don't have much conscious control over our heartbeat or temperature, when we are not thinking about our breathing, the brain stem does it for us. However, at any time, we can take control and make ourselves breathe faster or slower. In fact, we can even stop our breathing for various lengths of time.

In beginning meditation, one is taught to "follow the breath." But in fact, at first, what we do is *lead* the breath and become consciously aware of our breathing. We purposefully take a breath, follow it into our lungs, and let it flow around our body with various images or imagery. Then we consciously exhale and follow the breath out of our body.

As we repeat that practice and start to quiet and slow down, we begin to change our brain wave pattern from beta (awake activity) to the slightly altered state of alpha—the beginning of meditation and also the beginning of light sleep. In essence, this is our opportunity for spelunking into the deepest, most primitive part of our brain.

"Following the breath" really means that we stop *controlling* the breath. We become more aware of the breath as it moves from our conscious effort and gradually drifts back to the autonomic breathing of the brain. By following this process inward, we become calm, quiet, and altered. Also, by opening our minds and consciousness, we are allowed glimpses of the brain doing its true work.

These two meditations have served me well, both in my personal practice and in my professional work with others.

A Guided Meditation (in Technicolor)

- Choose a sacred place to do your meditation. This can be a predetermined place you've created in your home or garden, or a spontaneous place in nature.

- Take your time on each step or phase. Don't rush.

- Get into a comfortable, relaxed, seated position.

- Have the right attitude by coming into this process with **attention**. Be present and mindful of what you are doing without any outside (or inside) distractions.

- Set your **intention**, your reason for this moment's meditation.

- Choose a color you want to mentally surround yourself with during the meditation, e.g., sky blue, a yellowish atmospheric light, or green for grass or trees. It should be a color you can easily visualize with your eyes closed.

- Do a body visualization scan to determine any areas of stress or tension.

- Start a body relaxation process from your feet, moving up your entire body to your head. Release the tension and feel a nurturing, healing warmth until you have completely relaxed.

- Close your eyes. Many experienced meditators eventually leave their eyes slightly open.

- Perform the Wollman Meta4 Square Breath (see Chapter 20: Stress Management).

- After the last round, if you already have your own breathing technique, begin it. Or, if you don't have one, simply begin to breathe in and out without counting. Bring all your concentration to the in-breath and the out-breath. If possible, breathe in through your nose and out through your mouth. As we've discussed, the breath is one of the most important techniques to achieve a quiet mind. Follow the breath in and out for a few minutes, but slowly allow the breath to lead you and guide you into your meditative state. If at any point your mind starts wandering or if "monkey mind" sets in, return to focusing on the breath. When you are entering a meditative state, you will no longer need to concentrate on the breath.

- Remember that color you chose at the beginning? Picture the air you are breathing in as that color, entering your lungs and circulating out to every cell in your body. With each inspiration and expiration, picture this warm, healing, nurturing, colorful light turning the inside of your body into the same color you have imagined is surrounding your body.

- Now imagine that this exchange and movement of air in and out of your body is coming not only from your mouth and nose but also from every pore in your body.

- The color is now comingled inside and out. You begin to lose the confining boundary of skin—the boundary that previously determined "inside" and "out." You no longer recognize the confines of a body.

- Without confines, you may allow yourself to expand to the boundless reaches of the Universe. Stay in this space for as long as you can/want/desire.

- To begin the process of leaving the meditative state, return to awareness and consciousness by picturing all the energy and power of the Universe entering and concentrating within you.

- Repeat the Wollman Meta4 Square Breath.

- Do a postmeditation body visualization scan and compare it with your premeditation scan.

- Sense the harmony in Body, Mind, and Spirit.

- Did you achieve your **intention**?

- As you gradually, gracefully, and gratefully open your eyes, allow your new **attention** to enhance the rest of your day.

Another Guided Meditation

Here is another simple visualization/meditation I really like. I wish I could give proper credit, but I don't remember where I learned it. So, lacking a specific name, I will give credit to the Universe.

- First, visualize the universe and relish its expanse.

- Once you feel comfortable with your visualized universe, begin to experience yourself within that universe—your position, connection, and relationship.

- Luxuriate here for a brief eternity.

- Let go of the universe and reset. Now, simply visualize you—your being, your self.

- Next, begin to expand your realized self by eliminating all boundaries (see previous Guided Meditation).

- When you feel comfortable with your new, boundless self, endeavor to experience the universe within *you*. (Your eventual objective is to extinguish the boundaries between you and the universe.)

- Luxuriate here for a brief eternity.

Take your time with this; it can be repeated whenever you like. The more times you do this, the better you will get, and the more insightful the benefits will become.

Why Does Buddha Keep Smiling?

Sometimes, when I sit in front of my little Buddha statue, I meditate; sometimes I just think about things. Then, other times, I find myself testing Buddha.

Can I make him stop smiling by imagining things I might do? What if I steal from someone? He keeps smiling. What if I lie to a loved one? He's still smiling. What if I cheat a business partner? He's smiling just the same. I keep mentioning all sorts of things, and he keeps on smiling with approval.

Wait, he can't be smiling with *approval*, but he *is* smiling.

Maybe he knows that I am just testing him, or he sees that it is my karma to do "said thing." Perhaps he is smiling because he sees I have a few more lifetimes of learning but knows that I will eventually "get it."

Or maybe he is smiling because he loves me but is not *attached* to me. I am independent of him. I will do whatever I'm going to do, and he can still love me on a deeper level.

I get it! If I stop thinking I *own* anyone else, then I won't suffer loss if something happens to them. Then I can smile all the time like Buddha, and I can be happy with myself.

Wait. (Again.) I'm not supposed to think of the self, and neither is Buddha! So, why is he still smiling? It must be something deeper.

But right now I think it is best for me to start with the concept of no attachment to others. If that helps me smile, I might later begin to work on no attachment to myself.

KEEPING IT SIMPLE

Spirituality is not the same as religion. It is your personal communication and connection with the universe and noting your place within the cosmos.

Spirituality is about being grounded and centered.

It's important to have a daily spiritual practice as your guiding influence through your life's journey.

Mastering your spiritual practice during good times allows it to naturally arise during perilous moments.

Chapter Twenty-Two

Expansion: Balancing the Six Aspects

We discussed in Chapter 17: Nutrition that a cell on an agar plate, when placed near a toxin, will move away from it to avoid death. Remember? The same cell will move toward a nutrient to promote growth and ensure survival. In a sense, this is a form of contraction and expansion.

In the same manner, if we tune in to our bodies, it becomes apparent that things we don't like cause us to contract a little, and things we do like make us expand.

When we are aware of our Mission in life and are traveling that path, we get up each morning excited and expanding. When we have no Mission and nothing worth doing, we get depressed and don't want to get out of bed. We contract.

Every moment of our existence can be registered as a contraction or an expansion.

We have some control over this. When we meditate, for example, that might be the ultimate in expansion. We are expanding into the light and out into the universe.

The Gift of Mind and Consciousness allows us to connect to our body (the cells) and also to our Spirit.

What is the common link among the three? It is energy, in many forms. The Mind, the Body, and the Spirit all require various forms of energy (adenosine triphosphate, Qi, Prana) to enhance the function and relationship of each.

The Six Aspects of Optimal Health are the tools that provide and utilize energy. When they're used correctly, we expand. When they're disregarded or abused, the resulting imbalance causes us to contract.

The Mobius Strip

You may have noticed that I declared each aspect as the most important one. Did you write that off as either an error in editing or my patented "Goofy Glenn" humor? No. It wasn't a mistake or a joke.

Indeed, each singular aspect *is* the most important because they cannot be addressed separately. In practice, they are interdependent.

Don't believe me? If you're so clever, you tell me which one of the Six Aspects is the most important. Which one could be left out?

I'm waiting.

Still waiting.

You can't separate or prioritize them, can you? If you don't get enough sleep, you might not want to exercise. If you don't exercise, stress levels are affected. Stress levels may cause you to eat more, less, or the wrong food. When you eat poorly, you may not get a good night's sleep. And on and on it goes.

Would you rather be in a vicious circle or on a harmonious Mobius strip? Your choice.

Don't Ever Show This to Anyone

Occasionally, during certain shifts in the ED, it would feel as though we treated every baby in town during that one day. But at the close of the shift, when we looked at the actual logbook, we would realize we had only seen the usual number.

We also believed more crime and "weird things" happened during a full moon. This was also debunked by checking our logs.

Keeping a log can inform fallible perceptions. I encourage you to keep a logbook, a journal, or some other form of record of events so you can accurately look back on what happened during each day, rather than loosely recalling what it may have felt like. Also, it will show you important trends in your balancing process: in which areas you are improving and where you need more work.

I know it's not an easy habit to adopt. People I respected and cared about endlessly advised me to journal. I always fought it because I disliked—actually hated—writing (or at least the thought of it). It was easier for me to simply put some marks along a spectrum to record my progress.

So, for those of you who also dislike writing, let me share my template for a private log. In the modern age where we don't want to take a lot of time, it will satisfy the needs of a written journal and help you focus on some of the important things that will guide you in your pursuit of a balanced day.

If you are inclined to actually write a journal, my hat's off to you! That can be included and should be encouraged. But I have found that this log not only serves as a record, but also assists with decision-making in the moment. When you find yourself at a particular fork in the road, the choice you make can be positively influenced by contemplating where you later will be forced to place your mark.

In the following log, in addition to the Six Aspects of Optimal Health, I have also included a few daily practices that can enhance your life's path (giving proper credit and appreciation to Buddhism for the "Noble Eightfold Path," designed to liberate one from suffering).

To be fair, I should probably give a simple explanation of the additional categories not covered extensively in the Six Aspects—essentially, where to put the mark.

Good Thoughts: Where did your mind spend most of its time today: thinking about good, positive intentions, ideas, and issues, or negative, destructive, pessimistic concepts and beliefs?

Good Speech: Did you speak truth and express kindness and gratitude, or was there some gossip or inappropriate, unkind comments? Think of this category as an assessment of overall good verbal expression and communication. Good *listening* is also part of this category.

For a short story on how I learned a valuable lesson in mindful communication, visit **GlennWollman.com/ resources** and go to Guidepost 16—Watch the Road Signs: Share the Road.

Self-Care and Self-Appreciation: In Eastern thought, the first chakra (root chakra) expresses the necessity of meeting your basic needs before looking for enlightenment and other lofty pursuits. However, this isn't merely about brushing your teeth after every meal.

Optimally, in this category, you should have taken some time during the day to honor yourself and appreciate who you are. (Narcissists need not apply.) Suboptimally, did you denigrate yourself or deny your self-worth? Did you disregard your importance by taking care of others at the expense of your own health?

Care and Appreciation of Others: This is probably self-explanatory. Did you take time out of your day to help others, either spontaneously or in a planned way? If not, if today you were completely self-absorbed, give yourself a suboptimal mark and determine to make changes tomorrow.

Presence and Mindfulness: Are you in the moment, appreciating the moment?

For instance, suppose you are at a beautiful mountain lake with a waterfall, and a deer is drinking nearby. Is your mind on your taxes, a car repair, or what's for dinner? If so, you are not being present and mindful.

Likewise, if you are doing your taxes or preparing dinner and your mind is on a waterfall... well, you know where the mark should go.

Pain Management: You need to mark this category only if you are experiencing physical pain. If you are in pain, how well were you able to control it during the day? Was the pain disruptive or manageable? If you're not in pain... way to go! Congrats!

Balanced Day: This is not intended to be a mathematical total of all the prior categories. Instead, enter your subjective, general feeling about the day. Simply, did you feel an overall sense of balance, or did you become disproportionately engaged in any one concern to the exclusion of others?

The German philosopher Immanuel Kant believed that we are opaque and not transparent to ourselves. It is important to look into yourself as you fill out your log with honesty. If you knowingly enter incorrect information, it's time to look at an important pattern of behavior.

DAILY LOG: Your View of You

Date: _____

Suboptimal ⟵———————————⟶ Optimal

PATTERNS OF BEHAVIOR	☐	☐	☐	☐	☐	☐	☐	☐	☐	☐
NUTRITION	☐	☐	☐	☐	☐	☐	☐	☐	☐	☐
PHYSICAL ACTIVITY	☐	☐	☐	☐	☐	☐	☐	☐	☐	☐
SLEEP MANAGEMENT	☐	☐	☐	☐	☐	☐	☐	☐	☐	☐
STRESS MANAGEMENT	☐	☐	☐	☐	☐	☐	☐	☐	☐	☐
SPIRITUALITY	☐	☐	☐	☐	☐	☐	☐	☐	☐	☐
Good Thoughts	☐	☐	☐	☐	☐	☐	☐	☐	☐	☐
Good Speech	☐	☐	☐	☐	☐	☐	☐	☐	☐	☐
Self-care & Self-appreciation	☐	☐	☐	☐	☐	☐	☐	☐	☐	☐
Care & Appreciation of Others	☐	☐	☐	☐	☐	☐	☐	☐	☐	☐
Presence & Mindfulness	☐	☐	☐	☐	☐	☐	☐	☐	☐	☐
Pain Management*	☐	☐	☐	☐	☐	☐	☐	☐	☐	☐
Balanced Day**	☐	☐	☐	☐	☐	☐	☐	☐	☐	☐

*Only if applicable for physical pain

**A subjective, general feeling—not a total or summary of all categories

Personal Notes: _____

_____

_____

_____

_____

_____

Download a copy for your personal use at
GlennWollman.com/dailylog

So, what should you do with this daily journal?

Leave a blank copy out somewhere you can see it each morning after awakening and each evening before retiring. Record a subjective assessment of your performance in each category by checking the appropriate box on a scale from Suboptimal to Optimal.

You don't have to be overly critical or analytical about the placement of your marks. Remember, you are not showing this to anyone, so it is not being graded! (Relief for those of you who, like me, grew up wanting to get the A+ and extra credit.) Ultimately this is about self-awareness, self-improvement, and personal growth.

So, don't be anal (thank you, Sigmund). Sometimes, you may not even have to fill it out. Merely reviewing the categories will start your day off well, and you will make a difference with all those you encounter. But at the beginning, commit to using it for a week.

Here's an idea: Make 365 copies, one for each calendar day. (Okay, okay. You'll need one extra copy for Leap Day.) At the end of the year, notice the trends in each category. Design strategies to improve in the areas that need it and maintain your triumphant performance in the others.

But whatever you choose, *commit!* Just use it and see if it changes your day... and your life.

And, obviously, you are free to show this to anyone you want. (It's not like I'll show up at your front door to scold you.) But by not intending to show it to others, you can be more open and honest with yourself.

As time goes on and you are more comfortable with your openness, you might find yourself eventually sharing your thoughts with certain special people who will be interested—and supportive—in traveling this path with you.

Mind Shift

It's rather easy to see how cathartic journaling can be, but not if you dread doing it. Make this a fun exploration of your boundless self!

It became obvious to me as I began writing this: everyone should write their own book! Why not? Each of us has a unique story, and each of us is interesting in our own way. Think of a great title for your book and tell some stories as you travel your path, experiencing the world. Who knows? You may never show it to anyone, or it may be a best seller. (In which case, don't forget to list me in the acknowledgments!)

Health vs. Healing: Choose Your Priority

In looking back on the Six Aspects of Optimal Health, they can be focused in many ways on healing. But let me say this: they can be used even more beneficially to avoid the necessity of *having* to heal. Avoiding the need to heal should be our real health journey.

While practicing emergency medicine and running one of the only hospital-based integrative medicine programs in the country at the time, I had the idea to develop a facility that looked somewhat like a hospital (although more serene and happy) but was based on health rather than illness.

It would include areas for each of the Six Aspects of Optimal Health. For instance, one group would teach proper nutrition—how to grocery shop, cook, and eat. Another area would focus on stress management, teaching calming techniques of meditation and breathing exercises. And, speaking of exercises, another group would instruct in ways to exercise: Pilates, Qigong, tai chi, yoga, etc.

My idea was to call it a "Healthpital." Unfortunately, no one could stop laughing while trying to pronounce it, and it never happened.

When it comes to making healthy choices for life, you have to be introspective. Through each of the Six Aspects of Optimal Health, examine your mind. Decide if it is controlling you, or you are controlling it!

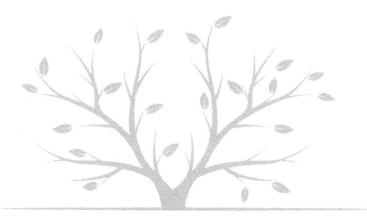

Let us decide on the route that we wish to take to pass our life,
and attempt to sow that route with flowers.
—Madame du Châtelet

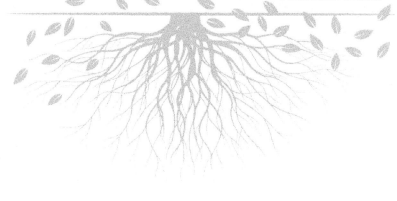

PART THREE

Your Path:
Navigating Health Care

Chapter Twenty-Three

Toll Roads

I have been in a unique position to observe countless individuals as they traveled their health-care paths. I recall the heavyweight boxer Mike Tyson once said, "Everyone has a plan for me until they get hit." Sadly, I discovered too many of us are just the opposite: we *don't* have a plan for our health until we get hit!

Over the years, I have grouped people into three general types of travelers based on the standard of care they set and provide for themselves. Now, I'm not referring to the way health insurance defines *standard of care,* but rather the way these individuals philosophically and concretely deal with illness or injury.

Which type of traveler are you?

The Passengers

This first group of people take little or no responsibility for their health. Wherever the road takes them, they will go. The majority of Passengers do not take care of themselves and, as a result, are unwittingly doing themselves harm.

If ill or injured, they stay on their path of avoidance until their home remedies and the "expert" advice from friends at work fail. When they ultimately are forced to enter the health-care system, they are generally in very poor health.

I've easily spotted these individuals during their emergency department visits. When I ask what medications they are on, the Passenger's reply is usually a shrug and an "Idunno." When I ask what surgeries they've had, their reply is "Idunno."

When treated, they do not develop any understanding of their medications or their illness and really don't care to know: "Idunno!" Passengers really don't want to take part in their own health or healing. They're along for the ride.

If the health-care path can be considered a toll road, the Passengers pay the highest toll.

The Navigators

These travelers map out their health care. They do their own research to understand their illnesses and injuries. Some of them head to the internet at the first sign or symptom and start "Dr. Googling" to come up with a differential diagnosis that would make a third-year medical student proud.

When they receive a diagnosis from their physician, they do additional research to become involved in their care and treatment. Navigators draft a road map for recovery, taking their responsibility as active participants seriously.

Navigators are also at a fork in the road. Some continue to be responsibly reactive to health-care concerns as they arise. Others choose to be more proactive by beginning to maintain their health in order to prevent medical maladies in the first place.

They are believers in "preventive medicines" such as childhood immunizations, flu vaccines, and antimalarial drugs. They schedule checkups, Pap smears, mammograms, and colonoscopies.

 To find out why I waited until I was seventy-two years old to have my first colonoscopy, visit **GlennWollman. com/resources** and check out Guidepost 11—Roadside Service: Rear Ended.

One caveat: I would argue they are under a slight misconception that those screening tests actually *prevent*

disease. Early detection can certainly halt a disease's progression (such as when we find a precancerous growth) or potentially can prevent a more serious disease from developing. But, obviously, by its very detection, the disease already does exist! We didn't prevent it at all. But, yes, we may have prevented it from getting worse.

Am I disparaging these screening tests? Au contraire! However, by the nature of the ever-changing guidelines for these tests, it's a good idea to speak with your doctor about what is right in your situation... which is exactly what health navigators would do!

For this group, the toll is reduced. Medical costs have a tendency to decrease. Granted, sometimes too much money can be spent on inappropriate or ineffective remedies and treatments. Overall, though, the more people that approach a balanced life, the better it is for the health system.

Although Navigators are on the right path, there is yet one more progression: a blossoming third group that I hope, with time, will become more and more prevalent.

The Drivers

These travelers, myself included, build on the practices of the Navigators. We know where we're going, but we've decided not to wait until we're ill to take action. We care for ourselves while we're well!

We have taken the wheel! We are conscious creators of our health and wellness. Our health-care toll is so greatly diminished, we feel as though we are on a freeway.

Our health habits are no longer focused singly on preventing illness, but rather on developing our higher consciousness.

Balance becomes our lifestyle.

True, we exercise to prevent heart disease, but also because the endorphins fuel a more positive mood, and a powerful body contributes to emotional strength.

We consciously eat more healthfully, sure, to prevent type 2 diabetes, but also to celebrate the sensory wonders of food or the joy of sharing a meal with a friend.

We use integrative therapies such as acupuncture and chiropractic. We do yoga, tai chi, or Qigong (among other practices) as forms of exercise and stress reduction.

Drivers know that we can't prevent all illnesses and injuries; some health-care road hazards are just unavoidable. We prepare for those unpreventable issues by keeping our bodies, minds, and spirits in the best daily health and best balance possible.

We do this utilizing the Six Aspects of Optimal Health. When illness or decline does inevitably occur, we are so well-practiced in using the Six Aspects that they easily become our tools to heal more effectively. (The Daily Log can be an integral aid in this practice.)

Rather than preventive medicine, I call this "preparatory medicine."

How do the three travelers approach health differently in a real-world situation? Let's look at a common health complaint: GI tract discomfort.

Passengers would first ignore any symptoms until the condition became serious. They might eventually receive a diagnosis of hiatal hernia, ulcer, colitis, GERD (gastroesophageal reflux disease), malignancy, or another of the problems it could be.

The science would provide medications to cure the condition—or at least hold the pathology in check. Sharp-edged instruments might be employed to remove the offenders. But the Passenger would do very little to enhance their recovery or avoid a recurrence. They're just a "ride-along."

Navigators would address the symptoms earlier. They would receive the diagnosis, actively participate in their treatment, and take responsibility for their outcome.

Drivers would perhaps have avoided the issue entirely by having changed their patterns of behavior before change was required. As part of our self-care, we believe in honoring ourselves, and we strive toward higher consciousness. We would have already endeavored to select higher-quality food, eat balanced meals, eat slowly, and chew more thoroughly.

Drivers appreciate food both as nourishment and as a gift. We look forward to our daily mealtimes with reverence rather than resignation, with an eye toward improving our digestion and improving the overall health of our GI tract.

Does that help make the difference in approaches clearer?

Okay, let's consider one last, more esoteric example: the case of a little girl who lost her father when she was only eight years old. At the time of his passing, she was overwhelmed with confusion and grief, and later developed abdominal pains.

Her caregivers were Navigators. After countless doctor visits, consistently negative workups, several diagnoses of psychosomatic issues, scores of prescribed meds, and many years, the patient finally was diagnosed with ulcerative colitis. She was then subjected to a seemingly endless cycle of steroid enemas, more medications, and surgeries removing more and more of her colon.

The road was long, hard, painful, and seemingly uncertain. Each surgery caused more scarring, more adhesions, and more pain, eventually leading to a colostomy bag. Horrific for a young woman trying to date and mate—just live her life.

Years later, as a mature adult, she was told yet another surgery was required. She instead chose to end her life. The road behind had been too hard, and the road ahead looked far too bleak.

What if during those early years, the eight-year-old had been cared for by a Driver? What if she'd been given the opportunity to address her issues along an integrative path?

For instance, a doctor of traditional Asian medicine (TAM), rather than continually looking at the symptoms, looks instead at the energy, as certain organs are well known to possess connections to particular energies.

Of course, if someone presents with determinable appendicitis, then naturally an appendectomy is performed. But in the absence of a tangible, physical cause for disruption and pain, the TAM doctor investigates the root cause.

This girl's physical symptoms would have been more closely examined in the context of her deep loss and despair. Her body would then be treated as a whole—as both a physical and a metaphysical being.

Insights from my colleagues at the former Santa Barbara College of Oriental Medicine suggested that the large intestine (which had so troubled this young lady) represents evacuation, letting go. A TAM practitioner would have helped her develop a process for letting go of her father. Perhaps the practitioner also would have addressed the lungs, which deal with grief.

If she could have taken control of her health care, what, then, could have been the possibilities for her future? Probably not a lifetime of doctor visits, persistent physical affliction, and eventual suicide.

You can see why I hope for a mind shift, and for this mindset to become more and more widely accepted. Perhaps someday, Drivers will emerge as the norm.

But for now, let me return to addressing the Navigators, those who generally travel the health-care path on a more traditional, yet many times "self-guided," tour.

Chapter Twenty-Four

The Self-Guided Tour

Intellectuals solve problems; geniuses prevent them.
—Albert Einstein

Some of my friends who have watched a lot of *Marcus Welby*, *Grey's Anatomy*, or *ER* are convinced the TV doctors have trained them to make informed medical decisions. (Insert my raised eyebrow here.)

While I generally suggest that they see an RD (real doctor) for an actual diagnosis, here are some important points to remember should you decide to throw on your proverbial lab coat and examine yourself following a minor injury involving bones, muscles, ligaments, tendons, or joints.

Remember earlier when I suggested you go to a bookstore or library and get a book on anatomy—one with big pictures and simple descriptions? If you haven't done that yet, let this serve as your reminder. If you can't be bothered to get in the car or order online, download an app!

This way, when and if you get hurt, you can see some pictures in front of you. (There's no need to memorize anything, unless of course it interests you to have an even deeper understanding of your body's anatomy.)

DIY (Do It Yourself)

In medicine, you'll recall that we first take a history followed by a physical exam. So, let's begin with taking your own history.

Understanding and documenting the answers will serve two purposes. You may discover, diagnose, and be able to treat your own problem. And if you do need to see a doctor, you will already have many of the answers about your condition, thereby participating in your own care by providing clearer clues for the physician.

- What was I doing when I first noticed the pain? (mechanism of injury)

- What movements make the pain worse? What aggravates the pain?

- What relieves the pain?

- Does it hurt only when I touch it or even if I don't touch it?

- Have I ever had this pain (or a similar pain) in the past?

- Give the pain a rating on an analog scale of zero to ten (zero being no pain and ten being the worst pain you have ever had).

- Describe the pain (e.g., burning, piercing, aching, tearing).

- Does the pain stay in one place, or does it radiate (spread) to other areas?

- Describe the action of the pain. Is it steady, constant? Or does it come and go? If you were making a graph of the pain, does it rise in intensity, then fall? Or does it spike (suddenly become intense)?

- What other symptoms come with the pain? Is there a temperature differential, numbness, tingling, etc.?

After taking this history on yourself (or on someone for whom you are caregiving), it's time for you to do a physical examination.

- Inspect (visually examine) the area of pain, looking for bleeding, deformities, swelling, discoloration, or lesions (e.g., abrasions, lacerations, punctures).

  ○ If it's an extremity, and you have an uninjured one on the other side, use the uninjured member as your role model—an example of what the injured extremity should look like. This can be especially helpful when you are in so much pain you forget what normal is.

  ○ If you see active bleeding, you should immediately apply pressure over the site. Depending on the amount of blood loss, get to an emergency department.

  ○ If you see a bone sticking out of your body—and you don't see a matching one on the opposite side—stabilize the area to prevent movement and head to the emergency department.

- Palpate (touch) the area very lightly to find a maximum point of pain.

  ○ During this process, you are also trying to define what specific part of the body is injured—for example, whether it hurts along a bone or within a muscle. As you become more familiar with the painful site, increase the pressure of palpation. This will help determine the seriousness and depth of the injury. Be very exact around a joint because they include muscles, bones, ligaments, and tendons. Refer to your anatomy book or app.

As you get to know your own body with more accuracy and gain understanding of movement around your joints, it will be easier to make your preliminary diagnosis.

○ In medicine, if we can't be sure of a specific diagnosis, we develop a differential diagnosis. That simply means we determine a few possible diagnoses, and over time, we will eliminate certain ones while possibly thinking of yet more. Likewise, you may arrive at several different conclusions. Determine the urgency of the most serious potential diagnosis and seek professional help accordingly.

• Move the area to help ascertain the extent of the injury and determine the next steps necessary.

○ We discussed this briefly in the chapter on Physical Activity. But this information is pertinent to any injury, not just those that occur in the gym.

○ If you sense that your injury is minor—not serious enough to warrant the emergency department—you can begin to stress the area slightly. The first movements of an injured joint should be PASSIVE. This means moving the injured part *without* utilizing the muscles normally used to move that part. For example, if you injured your left biceps muscle, use your right hand to bend your left arm at the elbow. If it hurts or causes pain, STOP. Don't go any further in your testing.

○ If passive movement doesn't hurt (or hurts only a little), then advance to ACTIVE MOVEMENT.

This tests the actual injured part. In our biceps example, try to bend your left arm without the assistance of your right.

- ○ If active movement doesn't hurt, proceed to move against resistance. In our example of the biceps muscle, this could be done by lifting a very, very light weight (say, a soup can).

- ○ Remember: do not do anything to increase the injury; you are only determining the extent of it.

- If you're not sure, then stop what you're doing and rest the area. Decide whether you can safely give it some time to recover on its own or if you need to be evaluated by a health-care professional.

It's a Long Road

When you are palpating bone or muscle as part of your self-diagnosis, remember that they are tissues made up of cells. So, when you have an injury, think small: you are actually injuring *cells.*

When cells are injured, certain physiological responses kick in to prevent further injury. You must do all you can to help your body in its healing process. Your body is what you revolve your physical world around. Deal with your acute injury appropriately and thoroughly to avoid its progression into potentially an even bigger problem: chronic injury—an injury that hurts all the time.

Chronic injury develops because while the body is trying to heal, many times you are too busy to let it. You choose to either ignore the injury ("Idunno"), "walk it off," or abbreviate the recovery period.

You don't listen to your own body.

Your cells then go into overdrive, continuing to react to inflammation, until finally you develop degenerative or chronic inflammation around your joints. That chronic inflammation eventually turns into arthritis or other problems resulting in pain and limitation of motion that will alter your daily life, possibly require medications or surgeries, and potentially even decrease your life span.

Don't risk wreaking havoc on the rest of your life by making bad long-term decisions based on short-term thinking.

KEEPING IT SIMPLE

Research your own body.

Learn a minimal amount of first aid.

While it may be fun listening to the other folks in the gym or to office coworkers who give you anecdotal treatments that a friend of a friend said worked well, *don't* necessarily add those treatments to your list of options.

When unexpected illness or injury throws an obstacle of sufficient gravity in your path, speak to your own doctor as soon as possible.

If you are referred to a specialist, trust them, and if you are having good success, don't complicate the issue with too many second opinions.

If, in the final analysis, you can't come to a decision, find a Medical Guide.

Chapter Twenty-Five

Navigating Difficult Roads with a Medical Guide

You only need to take care of the parts you want to keep.

—*Glenn D. Wollman, MD*

I f you choose to take the self-guided tour of the health-care path, it's up to you to take it prudently and judiciously. If you get lost or confused, or can't see the forest for the trees, that is the time for a Medical Guide.

A Medical Guide will closely examine the trees (your headaches, your heart palpitations, your fatty liver) while also taking you through the forest (everything concerning your life and your handling of each of the Six Aspects of Optimal Health). A Medical Guide is skilled at looking at both the small and the big pictures.

New-Drug Roulette

In earlier chapters, I've explained several ways in which a Medical Guide can be of importance to you along your path. But here is a particularly tricky road in traditional medicine that a Medical Guide can help you navigate—one that is becoming ubiquitous in advertising with you as the intended target.

No health-care path can be more confusing than one crowded with new "wonder" drug treatments. For instance, I often hear commercials soliciting participants for clinical trials of one drug or another.

On occasion, the trial is for a fatal condition, but more often, it is for a condition that is relatively well-controlled with current methodologies. I can understand taking a chance when you're out of choices. But the risk of taking treatments and/or drugs that have not yet been tested on large groups of people over a long period of time makes it akin to Russian roulette.

We Don't Know What We Don't Know (Even If We *Think* We Know)

One day as a third-year medical student on an internal medicine rotation, I was in a group of about eight classmates gathered to meet our new attending. He had amazing credentials: he'd just arrived from Harvard, was a leading authority in diseases of the liver, and had been the editor of the *New England Journal of Medicine*, one of the most prestigious medical journals in the world.

We were discussing a recently admitted patient and presenting the case to our new leader. It was an interesting and informative discussion. We instantly knew this new attending was going to teach us a lot, making us all better physicians in the process.

It was at this moment that one of the "brown-nosers" (you remember them, right?) quoted an article he had read in an obscure journal that slightly contradicted what the attending had just taught us. The usual groans ensued—although I must admit, the rest of us were briefly impressed that the brown-noser not only had found this article, but had presented it to the attending with such confidence.

As our peer was awaiting accolades, the rest of us were perched on the edge, waiting for our new Chief of Medicine's response.

Without hesitation, "Dr. Harvard" looked at our classmate and said, "Yes, I am familiar with that particular article, and I want to let you know that a new paper is going to be published in three months in an Australian medical journal, refuting everything that you quoted."

Wow.

Not only was he *familiar* with this obscure journal article, but he also knew of another paper that wasn't even published yet, from another part of the world!

I remember thinking at that moment, in silent self-query, "Is it ever possible to know all that we need to know to properly take on the societal responsibility for the health of people? How long will a fact remain a fact? How often during my career will I have to change my practice based on new facts that replace the old dogma?"

Every day we are exposed to new drugs, new treatments, and new theories on therapies. We're inundated with news of the latest antioxidant juice from a berry from South America, the newest treatment for an old disease, or a new way to get rid of fat and shape your body into something beautiful. Through technology, we have access to more information than ever before, and this is good.

YOUR PATH: NAVIGATING HEALTH CARE

However, in medical school and continuing through our careers, we doctors learned to be *discerning* in our reading and research. Who published the article? Was it biased? Who funded the research? Who benefited from its publication and results? Was it really a well-done study?

One dictum among the many that doctors hold is "Never be the first or last to use a drug or treatment." Don't be sucked in by brilliant marketing. Do your research. Learn about your own body and its needs. Something may be good for someone else but not for you—or vice versa. If you're considering a clinical trial, it is an especially good time to have a Medical Guide walk with you on the path.

One doesn't discover new lands without consenting to lose sight of the shore for a very long time.

—André Gide

"Boldly Go Where No One Has Gone Before"

One of my favorite aspects of the field of medicine is that it is a frontier made up of new drugs, innovative procedures, newly invented technologies, and ever-increasing knowledge. It makes it very exciting for those of us on a quest for understanding and provides great benefits for everyone subject to illness and injury.

But even those of us who love the frontier must chant a few mantras during our consideration of a clinical trial: risk-benefit ratio, double-edged sword, two sides of the coin, yin and yang, good and bad, pros and cons.

Under most circumstances, a clinical trial is considered when one has a life-threatening condition (for instance a type of cancer that is not responding to conventional treatments) and a sense of desperation sets in. They are also considered in situations that are not life-threatening but are severely affecting quality of life (such as fibromyalgia). And finally, there are those who consider clinical trials for minor conditions they find unappealing (like baldness).

This is really an important time for clear communication with your doctor, your loved ones, and your Medical Guide.

Here are some guiding thoughts I discuss with my patients:

- It is a trial. The drug on trial may not be completely proven, effective, or safe. The drug or treatment's safety and efficacy are what the trial will determine.

- Do your research on every aspect of the trial:

  ○ Who is conducting it?

  ○ Who is sponsoring it?

  ○ Is there a cost associated with the trial?

  ○ How conveniently located is the trial, and how many times will you have to go there?

  ○ What is the treatment schedule?

  ○ Which stage is the trial in?

  ○ How many different trials have been done for the same issue?

  ○ What are the results so far with other participants?

  ○ What are the benefits?

  ○ What are the risks?

- If time permits, do even more research.

- Consider the reality. Of course, one enters a clinical trial for the purpose of getting better.

But it is also good to keep in mind that if you choose to participate, you will also be benefiting future generations of those afflicted with similar conditions. That's a good thing. Thank you!

We Are Exactly Different

A Tibetan Buddhist monk and I walked into a bar.

(Not really, I just couldn't resist.) Let me start again:

A Tibetan Buddhist monk and I were having a discussion about acupuncture. Through an interpreter, I asked him whether he thought it was appropriate for acupuncturists to make so many claims regarding the multitude of conditions they could heal. My Western mind thought these claims discredited traditional Asian medicine because there were no double-blind, crossover, placebo-controlled studies to substantiate such claims.

I curiously awaited his answer.

He said, "Acupuncture can heal anyone, but not everyone wants to be healed."

That was a good lesson for me. His words guide me to this day as I make choices for my clients. Each client is an individual requiring individualized treatment.

We recognize ourselves as a specific species because we have many similarities to each other. On the other hand, each of us is unique. We are not exactly like our parents. We have different fingerprints. We have different blood types, intestinal biomes, and tissue types.

Each of us has a heart, a brain, and a liver. While on a cellular level those organs are all similar, each of our parts is unique in this world! Does everyone really have the exact same heart?

Therefore, to allow for the uniqueness of an individual, it seems quite logical to accompany Western medicine's treatment of the physical plane with additional individualized treatments for the patient's many planes.

The Humpty Dumpty Decision

In the emergency department, except for extreme circumstances like a decapitation, I believed everyone had the potential to be fixed. We would try until it became apparent that we couldn't succeed, and then we would stop.

Now, as a Medical Guide, when a new client comes to me, I assess their "Humpty Dumpty" status. Are they so broken that all the king's horses and all the king's men... you know the rest.

Going one step further, after I make my professional determination, I ask them if they see themselves as an H.D. (that's the clinical term for Humpty Dumpty).

Their answer helps to determine whether or not I can work with them—if we're in sync. Plus, it also gives me insight into how to guide them on their road to recovery.

The Medical Guide's Medicine Bag

Keep in mind, just as I don't do the surgery to remove a diseased organ (I send my client to the surgeon who best fits their needs), I also don't perform, say, acupuncture. Instead, I send my client to a well-chosen acupuncturist.

I serve as a guide to the diverse realm of healing modalities. I help people determine the appropriate specialists in allopathic medicine, and I also direct certain people to other healers and allied health professionals.

This is what I call combinatorial medicine. You may have heard others refer to it as integrative medicine, but I would like the word *combinatorial* to refer specifically to a practitioner who is more knowledgeable in Western medicine than most integrative medicine practitioners and ideally is a medical doctor or at least someone who can legally prescribe pharmaceutical drugs.

In order to know which specialty would be right for each patient, I have spent many years studying the various fields. I have taken many courses to learn about the alternative specialties. And I have traveled to various countries around the world to work with the indigenous healers directly.

Additionally, as I've mentioned, when I sustained my traumatic injuries and received multiple surgical procedures, I also involved other healing modalities in my recovery. So, I have not only learned about these specialties, I have personally *experienced* them with good results. (I also continue to employ various healing techniques to keep myself in balance.)

Each injury, illness, and recovery takes its toll. It is sometimes difficult to return to the way one was before the event. Although returning to your normal is always a good goal and motivator, the way you were before may have contributed to your illness or injury. As a Medical Guide, I look for ways to help you be different and *better* than you were before.

Because of my experience, counseling others has been a particularly fascinating process for me. I enjoy determining which individual will fit well with which singular healing modality or with which *combination* of specialties. Solving this puzzle requires me to understand the underlying belief systems of the clients as well as the methods in which they will most actively take part to permit the healing. It generally requires that the patient become a Driver, open to further developing consciousness of health.

Chapter Twenty-Six

Group Travel: The More, The Merrier

I am always looking for the best healing. After my traumatic motorcycle accident, I was left with a bad wrist fracture (requiring multiple surgeries), a complex pelvic fracture, and many other injuries. Suddenly, I found myself in full role reversal: as a patient in the very hospital I worked in.

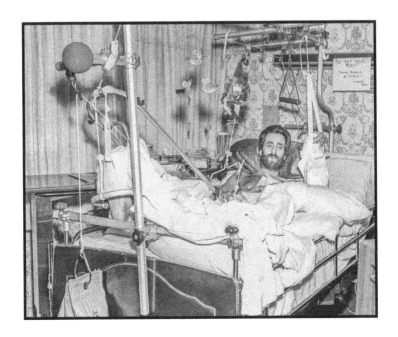

I was lying in my hospital bed, looking like the old proverbial injury cartoon. You know the one—with bandages everywhere, surgical pins in my bones, one leg and an opposite arm held in pulley systems, and traction keeping things stabilized. All this, so I could advance to even more extensive surgeries a few weeks down the line.

In the middle of the night, one of my favorite X-ray techs came in my room to visit. He was a unique individual from Haiti—smart, flamboyant, and good at what he did. We had always enjoyed conversations during our night and weekend shifts, and I appreciated his expert advice regarding special X-rays I should consider on specific patients.

On this particular evening, he had made sure to show up when no one else was around, and he asked if we could have a private talk. Of course! I had nothing else to do—and certainly nowhere to go—so I welcomed the conversation.

He then confessed to me that he belonged to a witches' coven and would like to bring them in to the hospital— quietly, of course—to surround my bed and work on me.

I trusted him and knew that this, first, would do no harm and, second, couldn't hurt! Partly wanting to experience the process and partly looking for anything to help me get through all this, I accepted.

I don't remember much of it, but I do know that I felt comfortable, nurtured, and safe. They never touched me, and they spoke softly in words I didn't understand— and I did not have to sell my soul or sacrifice an animal.

I don't recommend this road for everyone, but I do believe it is important for each individual to use all means available for health, treatment, and recovery. After multiple surgeries, multiple months in the hospital, a year filled with very painful physical therapy, chiropractic treatments, acupuncture and herbs, naturopathy, and my witches' coven, I was able to go back to work, happy again. Now, when asked what I think helped the most in my successful healing, I say, "All of it helped the most."

The Intangible

It's relatively easy to open up an abdominal cavity with a scalpel and point to an organ, or look under a microscope and examine a particular cell.

The esoteric, though, seems somehow easier to deny than the familiar. For instance, we can't "see" energy, yet we all recognize its tangible effects on us and, thereby, accept its existence and importance to us.

Anyone who has watched more than one episode of *ER* knows that invisible electrical energy, when applied properly to the chest wall using a defibrillator, can reboot an abnormally beating heart.

Light is another form of energy. The moods of people who live in areas with six months of winter are undoubtedly affected (from minor melancholy to full-blown seasonal affective disorder). Even if you live in a sunny area, after sitting indoors at the computer all day, how reinvigorating is it to be outside for a while?

Light also directly affects cells. Sunlight on the skin helps with the absorption of important minerals in our bodies. In our brains, light has an effect on the pineal gland's release of the hormone melatonin, which plays a major role in sleep and wakefulness.

But here, balance is the key. Portions of light energy—ultraviolet and infrared—can also do harm by damaging skin and eye receptors (even causing blindness in extreme cases).

Sound is another form of energy we don't deny affects us. Soothing sounds can improve appetite and aid in relaxation and sleep. However, just as with light, once again, balance is imperative. Extremely loud noises can destroy delicate cells and lead to hearing loss.

Haven't you used the effects of candlelight and beautiful music to promote a romantic interlude at some point in your life? Whether you realized it or not at the time, you were simply using energy for therapeutic purposes—well-balanced light and sound energy.

So, what about other energies? Energies we may be less familiar with than light and sound?

"Good, Good, Good, Good Vibrations"

I am about to border on the esoteric, and in fact, some of the next topics might even be considered ineffable. So, since words can't describe them, please close your eyes while I mentally transmit my thoughts to you.

(Just kidding.)

I do, however, ask you to suspend your disbelief for the next few paragraphs. If you have trouble believing in these, for the moment, just think of this as a fun hypothesis and follow along.

Many of the world's healing systems utilize some form of energy work. In traditional Asian medicine, the energy is called Qi (pronounced *chee*). It flows through various channels or meridians in the body. Acupuncturists use points along these channels to affect energy and bring about balanced flow.

The Mayan culture used similar points, but they referred to the energy as a "wind."

In Indian Ayurvedic medicine, the energy is called Prana, and it flows through chakras. Chakras are believed to be special centers located in and around the body, representing various portions of ourselves.

Yet other systems speak of various "subtle bodies" (such as auras, astral, emotional, and mental) surrounding each of us. They consist of and are affected by energy.

Imagine that each of these—with its own frequencies or vibrations—holds some connection to both the spiritual and the physical parts of the individual. If we are balanced in life, if all the bodies are in good frequency and harmony, we remain healthy and in various states of contentment or joy.

On the other hand, conflict, stress, or abnormal vibrations may be experienced as discord. These "bad vibes" may eventually make their way to the physical body, presenting themselves in the form of migraine headaches, chronic back pain, inflammatory diseases, and possibly even malignancies.

For instance, if someone has a stomach (gastric) ulcer, doctors generally prescribe antibiotics. Does that cure them? Do they need additional medications to prevent another ulcer? Does medication always prevent another?

The answer to each of these questions is "No."

Therefore, isn't it worth considering an additional part of treatment: a combinatorial analysis to discover the root cause of the underlying problem? It very well may be in one or more of the subtle bodies, centers, or energy meridians.

If you have trouble imagining these components of being, don't worry; the healers who practice these disciplines are very clear.

Imagination is the one weapon
in the war against reality.

—*Jules de Gaultier*

Alternative Highways

The importance of combinatorial medicine in prevention, preparation, therapy, recovery, and ongoing health cannot be overemphasized. Western medicine is excellent in diagnostics, trauma, and critical care, but it is neither perfect nor complete. This is why I've always tried to combine therapies to get the best results.

After surgeries for various issues, I have always used acupuncture, Chinese herbal therapies, homeopathic and naturopathic therapies, energy, and shamanic healing in some form—and have always had good results. So, I can attest to the fact that traveling your health-care path with a group is much more successful than going it alone.

Let me introduce you to some respected practitioners who have been involved in some part of my many healings and allow them to explain their specialties.

All these healing systems offer various ways to communicate with the cells. Whether herbs, poultices, needles, or drugs, the most effective treatment with the least risk of harm is usually the best.

Acupuncture

—Daniel Diamond, OMD (Doctor of Oriental Medicine), LAc, Nationally Licensed Acupuncturist

Acupuncture is a healing art, several thousand years old, and is a part of traditional Asian medicine (TAM). The acupuncturist inserts extremely thin sterile needles to affect the body's electromagnetic energy, referred to as Qi (pronounced chee). In addition to acupuncture, TAM therapies include electro-acupuncture, herbal medicine, massage and manipulation, moxibustion (dry heat), cupping, and advice about diet, lifestyle, and stress reduction.

Acupuncture points are specific sites where the Qi rises to the surface of the body. The electrical activity at these points can be measured with modern electrical resistance meters. The free flow of Qi throughout the body regulates all physiological activity. Therefore, pain and illness result from a disruption, blockage, or deficiency of the flow of Qi. Clinical studies have shown that the stimulation of acupuncture points causes alterations in heart rate, blood pressure, intestinal motility, blood chemistry, release of endorphins for pain control, and much more.

Many people feel a sense of deep relaxation during the treatment. Because the needles are extremely delicate, there is usually no discomfort when they are inserted (although occasionally a slight pricking sensation is felt). As few as four or as many as forty needles can be used. They are usually left in place for five to forty-five minutes, depending on the diagnosis and symptoms. The sensation while the needles are in place is often a dull pressure or nothing at all. The needles can have an electrical stimulus applied to them or can be manually stimulated or twirled.

Suction cups can be applied to the body to relax muscles and circulate blood that has "stagnated." These will sometimes leave a painless red or purple discoloration on the body for a few days. Herbal medicines may be prescribed in the form of a pill, powder, tea, poultice, or skin ointment. Massage and spinal manipulation (Tui Na) are sometimes also used.

According to Oriental medicine, the causes of disease are injury (trauma), poor diet, environmental and emotional stresses, heredity and genetics, excessive lifestyle (irregular sleep, recreational drugs, etc.), poor hygiene, and lack of physical activity. Bacteria and viruses are always present but are not the true cause of disease in TAM. Other factors will often weaken our immunity, allowing a bacteria or virus to proliferate within us.

The World Health Organization has found that acupuncture and Chinese herbs can be used for many conditions, including infections, allergies, depression, anxiety, and various internal, neurological, orthopedic, dermatological, obstetric, gynecological, and cardiological conditions.

The practice of acupuncture in the United States is licensed nationally, and some states require additional licensing examinations. Training programs in accredited private colleges of traditional Asian medicine granting master's or doctoral degrees range from twenty-five hundred to four thousand hours of education (depending on state and national laws) and take three to four years.

Esoteric Acupuncture

—Mikio Sankey, PhD, Licensed Acupuncturist, California

The main difference between Esoteric Acupuncture and the various traditional types of acupuncture theories that were developed in Asia is that Esoteric Acupuncture encompasses a much broader spectrum of healing and emphasizes the Wellness Stage versus the disease stages of the older systems. Esoteric Acupuncture can be utilized with traditional acupuncture theory to treat the physical body for ailments such as pain, insomnia, menstrual problems, digestive disorders, and a number of other physical ailments. But the focus of Esoteric Acupuncture is to harmonize and balance the center of the body in the areas known as chakras (especially the heart chakra) and to raise the level of one's consciousness.

Developing a greater overall awareness of life and understanding how everything affects the various body systems (physical, emotional, mental, and spiritual) will assist that individual to take more responsibilities in taking care of his/her life. People should not wait until a physical imbalance has taken hold to start making changes in their daily routine.

Since Esoteric Acupuncture does not focus on treating acute pain or chronic illnesses, the recommended treatment protocol is once every three to four weeks. Esoteric Acupuncture can also be used for "tuning up" the various body systems or for strengthening the overall immune system.

Modalities that complement Esoteric Acupuncture include tai chi, Qigong, the various types of hatha yoga, and especially meditation.

Esoteric Acupuncture is most beneficial to those individuals who are interested in expanding their levels of consciousness. Expansion of consciousness is the higher level of healing.

Traditional Asian Medicine

—JoAnn Tall, Doctor of Oriental Medicine

Traditional Asian medicine (TAM) is a comprehensive medicine that involves many modalities to achieve the same purpose: to create and maintain a state of emotional and physical health.

The underlying concept of this medicine is deceptively simple. In addition to all of the components of our body that Western medicine understands, TAM believes that there is an electromagnetic energy that courses through our system, nourishing and sustaining our physiological health. This energy is called Qi (Chinese) or Ki (Japanese).

Qi circulates throughout the body in specific pathways called meridians. Along each meridian are specific points at which the energy is more easily accessible and stronger. These are called acupuncture points. All of the modalities of TAM (acupuncture, acupressure, nutrition, breathing and movement exercises such as tai chi and Qigong, herbology, and lifestyle counseling) are geared to help this energy to flow freely and strongly throughout the body.

Acupuncture is the use of very fine needles to stimulate acupuncture points and meridians. Acupressure uses massage to stimulate the same points. Nutrition is the use of foods to correct imbalances in this energy flow. All breathing and movement exercises are designed to help maintain the strong flow of energy on a daily basis. Herbology is the use of herbs both simple and complex to achieve the same goal. And lifestyle counseling assists in determining how each person can adjust their work and home life to help them maintain this balance.

From these descriptions it becomes clear that the principle of keeping this energy strong, vibrant, and free-flowing is the prescription for—and the description of—good health.

This includes emotional health as well since there is no differentiation in this medicine between emotional and physiological health. If you are not emotionally well, then your energy is similarly disturbed; conversely, we can say that emotional dysfunction can be greatly helped by this medicine.

TAM may be used by anyone for any type of health problem, but common sense tells us that acute problems need to be dealt with by Western medical practitioners. It is also important that a Western diagnosis is ascertained, so that the best possible medical care can be achieved. TAM is a powerful and efficient complement to Western medicine; the smartest patient will use the best of both for optimal results.

It is important to understand that this is a complete medicine, used by millions for over two thousand years, and has a tremendous amount of medical research behind it. It is used for all types of diseases, yet it is most commonly used in the United States for pain of all types, addiction, and chronic degenerative disease.

In general, traditional Asian medicine has virtually no significant side effects; this makes it a treatment of choice either for stand-alone treatment or in combination with Western medicine.

Ayurvedic Medicine

—Khabir Southwick, TN, CAS, AP, AHP, PACE Provider

From the lush jungles of South Asia over the past thousands of years, a science of holistic healing has been methodically developed, studied, and put widely into practice. This science is called Ayurveda, which translates from its Sanskrit roots as "the science of life" or "science of longevity."

Over five thousand years ago, there are records of Ayurveda being practiced as a form of general health care by means of herbal medicines, dietary and lifestyle routines, yoga asanas, pranayama, and spiritual practices. These arts are all outlined in the Vedas, the oldest layer of wisdom teachings composed in the Vedic Sanskrit language, which originated in the ancient Indian subcontinent. Much of the wisdom of Ayurveda was passed down through generations of village people as an oral tradition through Sanskrit hymns, which were later recorded in writing.

Through meticulous study of each plant, mineral, and substance their fertile environment provided, these ancient people were able to document the actions of many herbal substances on the human body and their uses in all types of ailments they encountered. It was observed, in their closeness to nature, that all things in this world contain the five elements of ether (space), air, fire, water, and earth. Over time, they understood a form of intelligence that directed the movements and manifestations of the elements, and they called these intelligent forces the three "doshas," named vata, pitta, and kapha.

In modern times, people are easily able to research their Ayurvedic "body type" online and find lifestyle guidelines for vata, pitta, and kapha. But in the ancient practice of

Ayurveda, these doshas were seen as together being the forces which are in place to maintain all biological life.

Vata, the dosha that governs ether and air, is understood as the force of all movement in the universe, from cell division to continental shift. Vata is known best by its qualities of cold, dry, light, and mobile. We usually see vata-dominant people physically as being thin or "light," tending toward underweight, as well as very dry and dehydrated. These people are easily cold in temperature, tending toward low blood pressure and poorer circulation. Their most common character trait is their creativity and active mind, which often leads them to have lots of projects going on at once, with many creative thoughts and ideas. A weak point for these people is a tendency toward stress, anxiety, and overthinking. Overall, vata types are outgoing, friendly, and fun-loving people.

Pitta is the dosha that relates fire and water, whose energy originates from the sun and, thus, is the principle of heat and metabolism. This dosha is known by its qualities of hot, sharp, and mobile. Individuals with dominant pitta dosha tend to be strong, assertive, goal-oriented people who make great athletes. These are people who have a higher body temperature physically, a very strong appetite for food and for life, and a tendency to be "hotheaded," angry, and hypercritical. Pitta-type people are usually highly confident and charismatic, with their main weak point being their tendency toward developing pain and inflammation.

Kapha is the dosha that governs the elements of water and earth, the structure of which the other elements are moving in and through. We can understand kapha through its qualities of being heavy, slow, soft, cool, oily, and fluid. People who are dominantly kapha in their constitution have a tendency to be heavy or gain weight easily, slow to rise in the morning, slow in their speech, and usually very patient and mild-mannered. They are soft in their mannerisms and dealings with other people, and *physically cool in temperature. Kapha-type people tend to have oily skin and are prone to swelling due to water retention. These people are very nurturing, caring, and loving toward others. People with dominant kapha dosha tend to have the fewest health problems, though a main concern would be the tendency toward slow metabolism and excessive weight gain.*

These three doshas each have their importance and functions in the maintenance of the human body. When they are in balance, we find ourselves having regularity in our bodily functions and a general sense of peace and happiness in our lives. All too easily, though, one or more of the doshas can become imbalanced. When left untreated, these imbalances manifest into diagnosable diseases and health problems. When we are able to clearly understand the "tri-doshic theory," we are then able to begin understanding our own physical constitutions and those things that will bring us back into balance.

In the practice of clinical Ayurveda, practitioners utilize ancient diagnostic methods including the art of reading a patient's pulse, as well as observing the state of their tissues and asking them specific questions. These diagnostic methods take years to master, and eventually allow the Ayurvedic practitioner to thoroughly understand not just the patient's original state and their imbalances, but also the pathology that took place to manifest their health problems.

The Ayurvedic pharmacist, when well studied, well practiced, and with many herbs available, is able to design a protocol of herbal treatments that will address the imbalances a patient has, as well as design for them a diet and give them lifestyle guidelines that will bring them closer to a physiological state of harmony and balance.

Osteopathic Medicine

—Timothy T. Schultz, DO, CNMM

The American Association of Colleges of Osteopathic Medicine (AACOM) leads and advocates for the full continuum of osteopathic medical education to improve the health of the public. Founded in 1898 to support and assist the nation's osteopathic medical schools, AACOM represents all thirty-seven accredited colleges of osteopathic medicine—educating nearly 33,800 future physicians, 25 percent of all US medical students—at fifty-eight teaching locations in thirty-three US states, as well as osteopathic graduate medical education professionals and trainees at US medical centers, hospitals, clinics, and health systems.

Osteopathic medicine, like allopathic (Western) medicine, has gone through several "structural changes" since its inception in 1892. The practice of osteopathic medicine started as a vision of A. T. Still, MD, as a practice of American frontier medicine. It is based on the tenets of structure/anatomy affecting function/physiology of the individual person with medical symptoms. In Still's paradigm of medicine, disease state was secondary to treating the patient; found within the body was the patient's own "healing" response. (The immune system had yet to be discovered.)

The philosophy was born at a time when pharmaceuticals, even aspirin, had not been discovered, and "medications" of the time were mostly detrimental to the patient's chances of survival/recovery. The osteopathic physician made a physical diagnosis based on touch—paying attention to the patient's specific anatomy and physiology while reasoning that through osteopathic manipulation/adjustment we improve the ability to fight disease and improve function.

The study of anatomy was key to the reasoning behind disease and health. As an example, the Spanish flu epidemic of 1918–19 killed between fifty million and one hundred million people worldwide, with nearly one-third of people infected. The mortality rate (2.5 percent in the United States) among patients treated by osteopathic physicians was significantly lower than for those treated by MDs.

Although this philosophy is still pervasive in US osteopathic medical school teaching and training, it has been placed in the background of a fully licensed physician who practices in an enlarging and demanding, specialty-driven health-care paradigm. Currently 25 percent of physicians in training (125,000 total) are in osteopathic colleges (33,800). Many practicing osteopathic physicians currently relegate osteopathic manipulation to its historic merits without following its original tenets or using any specific manipulation in "treating disease" (cultivating health).

In distinction, European osteopathic programs that do not grant full medical licensure have also grown exponentially and keep the physical medicine priority in patient care. The European system does not, however, train its students to prescribe medication or perform surgery, nor does it provide a full spectrum in the study of disease. There is an obvious advantage and disadvantage to each system of training.

Currently, a board-certified medical specialty exists within the practice of osteopathic medicine: neuromusculoskeletal medicine. It emphasizes the importance of simultaneously diagnosing and treating the body with osteopathic evaluation and treatment modalities, and then, based on a treatment plan specific to the patient diagnosis, implementing care. Addressing structural or anatomical variance from trauma, birth, infection, or disease process becomes the priority of neuromusculoskeletal practitioners.

With the study of anatomy in mind, the practitioner uses anatomy as a specific guide while palpating variations of "normal" tissue directly in the patient. These variances are accessed and altered in real time through neurologic and muscular "feedback" from the patient's physical response to treatment. The osteopathic physician, skilled in neuromusculoskeletal management, is "triaging" tissue changes and anticipates those that affect vascular, nerve, ligament, and joint function. Supporting postural stability that may result from the supportive links of "comingled tissues" can be of significant therapeutic benefit and can even address some of the body's inherent mechanisms of healing, which, in turn, address manifestations of disease.

The practice of osteopathy is inherently patient-centered, responsive to the individuality within the person seeking medical care. Its vision is not limited to the body but includes both mind and spirit. Osteopathic care addresses the nature of the human being, who expresses suffering as triune: body, mind, and spirit.

Chiropractic

—Steve Blaut, DC

What is chiropractic?

Doctors of chiropractic employ a method of healing that gives particular attention to the structural and neurological aspects of the body—particularly the spine—in the treatment and prevention of disease. The clinical examination of the patient is similar to that done by the allopathic physician, and the same diagnostic testing is employed in the evaluation of disease. Subluxation is a common cause of pain, and if treated correctly, the patient's complaints typically resolve quickly and proper function returns.

When is chiropractic appropriate?

First, the chiropractic physician performs a comprehensive diagnostic evaluation to rule out serious pathology. If biomechanical faults are identified—spinal or extremity joint dysfunction—then the patient is a good candidate for a course of chiropractic treatment to reestablish proper mechanical function. Patient involvement in exercise and other home therapies should be recommended by the chiropractic physician to shorten healing time and maximize long-term results for the patient.

Why chiropractic treatment?

Acute traumatic or chronic spinal and other joint pain typically responds well to chiropractic care. Subluxation is the main cause of pain in most acute and chronic joint complaints; chiropractic treatment is directed to restore proper function in the human body. Chiropractic is unique in its approach of treating the patient's illness from a biomechanical restorative approach without drugs. As chiropractic medicine has evolved, medical and chiropractic physicians work in concert to restore function to the patient, maximizing health and vitality.

Bodywork

—Katie Mickey, massage therapist

Bodywork is a bridge to harmony and balance within the body/mind. From the particle perspective, bodywork employs assorted mechanical manipulations to various tissue layers for the purpose of enhancing function, posture, and behavior. From the wave perspective, bodywork blends skillful touch and intuitive sensing for the purpose of activating the healer within. Bodywork as a therapeutic modality encompasses a broad range of techniques and approaches to effect positive change in the body/mind.

Bodywork has its roots in traditional medicine. Hippocrates, the father of Western medicine, employed bodywork as a principal modality. In the early eighteenth century, Per Ling developed Swedish massage to cure his rheumatoid arthritis. Several decades later, American medical pioneers such as Harvey Kellogg offered massage in spa-type retreat settings to treat tuberculosis and other assorted maladies.

Today, bodywork is the treatment of choice by millions of wellness consumers who are actively generating their state of well-being, peak performance, and body/mind integration, as well as those seeking relief from pain and disease. Today there are hundreds of styles of bodywork practiced in various cultures and settings throughout the planet for the purposes of healing and stress reduction.

Bodywork's benefits can be felt on several levels of the body/mind. The specific effects that arise from any treatment session are a by-product of the techniques utilized and how they are administered (in terms of depth, pace, rhythm, direction, and duration), as well as the presenting patterns within the recipient and the practitioner.

Within the eleven body systems, bodywork can activate the parasympathetic nervous system, increase the circulation of fluids, flush waste products from tissue, relax hypertonic muscles, soften connective tissue, increase range of motion in joints, stimulate digestive and eliminative function, release "feel-good" endorphins, heighten sensory awareness, and enhance vitality.

Within the emotional body, bodywork can release heavy feeling states, unwind trauma stored within the tissue as the fascia releases, and induce states of joy and lightness of being.

Within the mental body, bodywork can quiet the mind, reframe perceptions of self, and transform limiting beliefs and behaviors.

Homeopathy

—Lauri Grossman, DC, CCH, RSHom(NA)

Homeopathy is a system of natural healing that uses ultra-low-dose medicines to strengthen the body and to prevent disease. It can be used to alleviate physical, emotional, or mental symptoms when they are acute (like colds, sore throats, and headaches) or when they are chronic (like asthma, anxiety, and insomnia). For over two hundred years, homeopathic medicines have safely assisted individuals around the world. And for over one hundred years, the FDA has regulated their use in the United States.

Homeopathy was founded by a German physician, Samuel Hahnemann, who discovered a way to prepare natural substances so that they could stimulate the body's own healing abilities. He based his work on the Law of Similars: using micro amounts of substances that cause certain symptoms in healthy people, to cure those same symptoms in unhealthy people. (This is a similar principle to that underlying the use of allergy shots for people with allergies.)

When compared with other forms of medicine, homeopathy stands out because it is gentle and not associated with harmful side effects. To relieve symptoms, it stimulates the healing mechanisms of the body. So, problems can be cured (and not suppressed), and individuals can become more resistant to disease after treatment. What's more, there are over six hundred published research studies in the field, and homeopathy continues to be one of the least expensive forms of medicine. (When compared with conventional care, homeopathic services are 20 percent of the amount and prescriptions are only 10 percent.)

Reliable websites for more information include **homeopathycenter.org** and **hri-research.org**

Naturopathic Medicine

—Robert I. Reynolds, PhD, NMD
Author, The Will to Health: Inertia, Change & Choice

Naturopathy, as a modern system of medicine, has flourished in frontier towns and wide-open spaces. The "nature cure" and homeopathic movements that began in Europe needed room to grow and an environment close to nature. As such, nineteenth-century America and twentieth-century Canada and Australia welcomed an approach to medicine that emphasizes the individual patient's ability to achieve health by improving his/her interactions with the environment.

In practice, this means taking in clean air, water, sunlight, and food, while discharging unwanted toxic waste. Therapy involves removing factors that are disturbing a healthy balance while establishing vital physical and psychosocial boundaries.

Naturopathic medicine combines Western knowledge of medical science with traditional healing techniques and a homeopathic philosophy. Naturopathic physicians are the only primary care physicians trained in a variety of natural therapeutics: clinical nutrition, botanical medicine, homeopathy, acupuncture, manipulation, hydrotherapy, exercise, and hypnosis. Naturopaths combine and tailor these treatments to the needs of the individual, based on an assessment of the underlying cause of an illness and a philosophy that views the patient as an active participant.

Despite the wide range of treatment modalities available to the naturopath, this school of medicine is most clearly distinguished by its philosophy. There are six underlying principles:

- *The Healing Power of Nature*
- *Identify and Treat the Cause*

- *First Do No Harm*
- *Doctor as Teacher*
- *Treat the Whole Person*
- *Prevention*

The underlying philosophy has its roots in the medicine of Hippocrates, Tibb (Middle Eastern), Ayurveda (Indian medicine), and homeopathy. The body-mind complex is seen as continually exercising its ability for self-healing. The physician's role is to stimulate and support this natural process in as gentle a way as possible. Ultimately, the physician serves to educate, empower, and motivate patients to take responsibility for their own health.

Naturopathic medical colleges are four-year postgraduate schools with admission requirements comparable to those of conventional medical schools. Following completion of pre-med courses, naturopathic medical students take three thousand hours of academics and twelve hundred hours of supervised clinical internship, and national board examinations in basic and clinical sciences. Naturopathic doctors are licensed as primary care physicians in a growing number of states in America and certified in Canadian and Australian provinces.

Sangoma or Inyanga Medicine

—David Cumes, MD

To most Westerners, indigenous African healing techniques are at best puzzling and at worst smack of sorcery. The West is replete with technological wonders. Our communication network is a veritable marvel with the likes of satellite phones, fax machines, and the internet. Yet ancient African wisdom has a lot to teach us about communication. There is a realm of spirit, but there is also a veil that must be penetrated if we wish to communicate with this potential source of guidance.

Most Westerners do not have the techniques to pierce the veil; sangomas do. Sangoma medicine is very practical. If you have lost a cow, the inyanga can throw the bones and tell you where to go and look for it. The techniques are evidential and have stood the test of time.

Sangomas and inyangas work with diagnostic and therapeutic methods just as we do in the West. Diagnosis is made either through the medium of spirit possession, through the divining bones, or through the dream-time.

In the case of spirit possession (called trance-channeling in the West), the guiding spirit possesses the body of the healer and imparts the information directly through the sangoma, sometimes even talking in "tongues." It is the sound of the drum that calls the spirit into attendance, and the word sangoma comes from the Zulu word for a drum.

In the case of the "bones" (which are not all strictly bones), the spirit manipulates the energy field so that when they fall, they can be read in an intelligible fashion. The diviner is the messenger for the voice imparted by the spirit world.

To some healers this veil is most permeable during sleep, especially in the early hours of the morning, when the ancestors may impart "instructional" dreams to the inyanga. Sangomas often dream about their patients before they visit and may even dream of specific plants to rectify patients' particular problems. These revelations of the night are a crucial and vital part of the healing repertoire.

In both cases, the diagnostic information is not localized in space and time. Both bones and dreams can speak to the present, past, or future, and the guiding spirit can tell the client what is happening to a loved one far away. The bones are reading the waking dream that is the patient's life, and interpretations are understood in metaphor much like dream interpretations.

Treatment is dispensed with the help of plant medicines (sometimes mixed with animal products) that are administered in numerous ways such as ingestion, steaming, bathing, by enema, by incision, etc. Powerful rituals (including animal sacrifice) are also made on behalf of the patient to invoke the necessary healing from the ancestors.

Sangomas help, heal, and work in the light on behalf of their people, but dark messages are also propagated through an impartial cosmic "field." Witchcraft and sorcery also occur, since there can be no light without dark—no rose without a thorn. Sangomas must know how to deal with witchcraft and how to counteract it.

Good News and Better News

In medicine today, as you lie in your uncomfortable hospital bed, stylishly clad in your hospital gown, the physician says, "We have good news and bad news. You have cancer, but we are lucky to have caught it early."

Detecting cancer after it has materialized is supposed to be the good news?

Unfortunately, it is very possible that by the time cancer reaches the physical body *in any form*, we have actually caught it *late*.

If this is the case, it seems even more important to pursue harmony within all of the bodies—physical, subtle, emotional, etc. This puts pressure on the various healing systems to work together to develop technology to quantify energy and vibrations in the subtle bodies.

This will be *true* combinatorial medicine.

In the future, my hope is that we will focus equally on frequencies within the body and measurements of those frequencies to detect abnormalities and indicate whether the body is in a state of imbalance—just as we now use vital signs (blood pressure, pulse, temperature, respiratory rate, and pulse oximetry).

If we were able to find a "normal" range of vibration and frequency, diagnostics would tell us when something subtle was out of balance. We could then do further studies to determine the cause and conclude a treatment perhaps involving energy frequency modification.

Maybe someday we will actually be able to say to our patients, "We have good news and *better* news. We found something in your emotional body that needs healing, and we can prevent a future physical consequence!"

Possibly at some point in the future, this integrative approach will no longer be called combinatorial medicine.

It will just be called *medicine*.

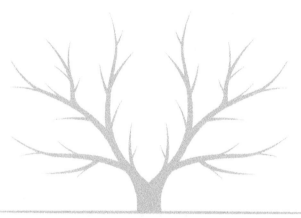

Everyone has two lives. The second one
begins when you realize you have only one.
—author unknown

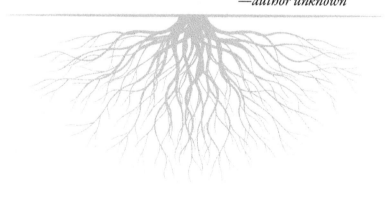

PART FOUR

The Path of Questionable Existence: A Dead End or a Cul-de-Sac?

Chapter Twenty-Seven

Decline, Dysfunction, and Death: Having Fun along the Way

From the moment of conception, our usual fetal trajectory begins with growth, but dysfunction, decline, and death quietly lurk in ever-present competition.

As the umbilical cord is cut and the physical connection to the mother is permanently severed, a first of many breaths is taken. This moment declares itself: "I am alive. I am me (even though I don't yet have the concept of 'me')." The assumption is that growth and development will follow—excluding genetic disorders, traumatic events, and critical illnesses. At this point, and for at least forty to fifty years, most of us remain in that state.

But then it happens. We hit the top of the bell-shaped curve, and we begin our downward slope of decline until dysfunction and death prevail. Sometimes it's not a pretty sight.

The best defense is to practice lifelong preparatory medicine. It may slow down the aging process—increasing the time it takes to get to the top of the curve and the decline phase.

On a positive note—assuming we are not obliterated by a nuclear attack, a large asteroid, a supervirus, an antibiotic-resistant bacterial strain, or an environmental collapse—there is always the possibility we might eventually evolve into a new and improved version of *Homo sapiens*.

Perhaps *Homo virtualis*? Or *Homo artificialis*? What do I mean? My concept is, over time we will have not only organ transplants, but also new technological organs that can be repeatedly replaced. Artificial intelligence will be entered into our consciousness. At that point, we may never die; we will simply need upgrades and replacement parts.

In this future, you won't need to follow any of my ideas and advice for preparing for death. You'll just have to make sure your "human parts warranty" remains current.

But for now, we need to accept and plan for decline, dysfunction, and eventually our death. Our approach, however, does not need to be dark or maudlin. As the chapter title says, let's continue to have fun along the way.

 For a personal story of mind shifting, visit **GlennWollman. com/resources** and read Guidepost 6—Road Games: The Instrument Panel and Guidepost 20—The Souvenir Shop, if you're interested in seeing results.

Chapter Twenty-Eight

Gawkers and Gawkees

*A good traveler has no fixed plans
and is not intent on arriving.*
—*Lao-tzu*

The "green flash" takes place when the sun is almost entirely below the horizon—either at sunrise or at sunset—when only a small portion of the upper rim is visible. Due to an optical phenomenon, the sun and a portion of the sky will appear green. Because I am a night person, sunsets are my preferred time to hunt for the green flash and try to photograph it.

I have seen it only once but never captured it with my camera.

My entire life in medicine included looking into the eyes of every body I examined: beginning with my cadaver and moving through newborns, children, adults living, adults dying, those brought back to life, and those who were dead. Of course, I inspected the anatomy of their eyes: orbits, eyelids, pupils, white and colored portions, and even deeper into the physical structure with optical instruments and scalpel.

I also looked for—and found—a difference: an emanating inner light (a quality) that would shine in the healthy, dim with the ill and dying, and be absent in the dead.

Because of my unique specialty, I delivered many babies, cared for people in various stages of life (with a wide variety of illnesses and injuries), successfully resuscitated people, and witnessed death at its very moment.

Could there be a green flash equivalent with the light coming on at birth (sunrise) and going out at death (sunset)? For years, I searched. It was much more difficult—and possibly impossible—to see at birth, but maybe I could see it at death.

Finally, I saw it once, and then a second time a few years later. I not only saw the light leave the eyes, but both times it appeared to rise or fly off.

From the beginning of human life, we have tried to peel away the veil to witness the face of death. Most individuals don't have many opportunities to witness someone during their actual moments of dying. Despite a lack of firsthand experience (or maybe because of it), humanity retains an unrelenting fascination with death.

For instance, go to a sporting event where people have paid thousands of dollars for first-rate seats. More than likely, every one of them would turn around to watch a fight in the stands—even if Ali and Liston were in the ring duking it out. Everyone went to see the blood and gore! It doesn't matter whether it's in front of them in the main event or behind them as fans disagree over a reserved seat. The fascination with possible injury to the point of death persists.

Another example is in the form of a personal admission: one thing that really irritates me is being stopped on a freeway. Fully stopped. Even if I am going one mile an hour, I am relatively okay. But when the freeway becomes a parking lot, I tend to get frustrated. (This a perfect time for the Wollman Meta4 Square Breath technique that I discussed in the chapter on Stress Management.)

But, invariably, I discover the cause has been a car accident, although the damaged cars have already moved to the side of the road! So, the reason for the insufferable traffic jam is not a *physical* blockage, but instead the cause is *gawkers* slowing down for a chance to see "blood, gore, and death." Let's just say that *really* tests my neuroendocrine system.

As the gawkers rubberneck to stare at the accident, subconsciously wondering if they will witness a death moment, they are in danger of causing (or at least being part of) another accident themselves! In the blink of an eye, they risk transitioning from gawker to gawkee—possibly offering someone else the opportunity to view a death moment. All in the name of fascination with death.

What is the key to extinguishing our endless fascination? Eliminate—or at least decrease—our fear. Take the concept of death to a comfortable level within our own psyches. Can you imagine a society of non-gawkers? Wouldn't life be better?

Chapter Twenty-Nine

What Are We Teaching Children about Death?

To realize how short life is,
you must live a long time.

—*author unknown*

As is the case with many lifelong fears, fear of death begins in childhood. There are many versions and many descriptions of death: mythological, religious, and philosophical. But perhaps some of the most impactful are the views of death contained in nursery rhymes, fairy tales, fables, and even lullabies.

Pray tell, how are children supposed to fall asleep to a lullaby chronicling babies left in unsafe conditions who may possibly die at any moment? You think I'm exaggerating, don't you?

Remember:

When the bough breaks, the cradle will fall,
And down will come baby, cradle and all.

Nice.

Traditional children's prayers are no better. "If I should die before I wake..."? What a thought to instill into a child, especially right before bedtime!

Is reading them a story a better choice? Not necessarily. The Brothers Grimm were certainly grim. They made their mark writing bedtime stories that convinced children evil was out to get them, and death was lurking around every corner. Snow White's poison apple and Hansel and Gretel's push into an oven by a wicked witch are just two fear-inducing examples.

So, okay. Enough of the books. Let's take the kids to the movies instead. Or maybe not. Children's films are replete with dead parents: *Tarzan*, *The Lion King*, *Bambi*, *Cinderella*, *The Little Mermaid*, *Finding Nemo*... the list goes on. Is it any wonder many children grow up with an indelible fear that their parents could suddenly die?

So, what are we teaching our children about death? As we ponder these examples from our childhoods, it's fair to ask, "How did any of us grow up normal?" That's my point. We didn't. We're the ones gawking on the freeway and turning to watch fights.

If we want to foster a future world with less fear and less of an unhealthy fascination with death, care should be taken with the stories we offer in childhood. Perhaps, when our children can't avoid certain stories that are ingrained in popular culture, we can take steps to add a bit of healthy context.

 For more thoughts, insights, and wisdom to consider when raising children, visit **GlennWollman.com/resources** and check out Guidepost 4—Travel Companions: Baby on Board.

Chapter Thirty

Hello Muddah, Goodbye Fido

We will all lose our parents, so there is little point trying to either whitewash or avoid the subject. It is a natural progression of our existence; there is no excuse for not facing it head on.

No matter on which side of the equation you find yourself, don't leave anything unsaid. If you are not one given to lengthy conversations, at least say the important words "I love you" throughout life, and especially before death.

If you want to gain wisdom about death—or teach your children through an experiential lesson—keep a pet, sit back, and wait. (Note: I say "keep," not "own." We really don't *own* anything, especially animals—and clearly, we don't own cats!)

You'll have a lot of fun along the way. But, unfortunately, we *Homo sapiens* have a longer life span than most of the species of pets. (So, if you intend to provide a relatively immediate lesson, opt for a goldfish, not a tortoise, or a parakeet instead of a parrot.)

We learn to love our pets on many levels and at many depths. Eventually, however, something is going to happen to them. That eventuality presents tough lessons, albeit really good ones about life and death as well as dying and loss.

When it occurs, explain death to your child in keeping with your philosophy.

We shouldn't make up stories that are sugary or whitewashed. You may feel you are being kind in the short run, but evading the subject doesn't teach them anything useful for their lives going forward. A pet's death is the opportunity to say, "This is going to happen to all of us. It's natural, and it's okay."

The explanations you give will determine whether your child grows up with an irrational fear or a healthy understanding of death. Choose your explanation wisely, with the future in mind.

Chapter Thirty-One

No Need to Be Tense about Past, Present, and Future

Usually, we think of history as things that have already happened and are now in the past. The other day, I heard someone use the expression "as history unfolds." To me, that implies that history is actually in both the present and the future—it just needs to be "opened and exposed."

But then I listen to many philosophers, gurus, and mind leaders telling us to remain "in the present." "Be here, now." "Be mindful."

This made me wonder, *when* is the actual present?

The moment you think of the present, it is already in the past. If you are waiting for the present to appear, it elusively remains in the future.

I don't think we should live in the future (that tends to cause anxiety for some), nor do I think we should live in the past (as that can cause depression for many), and as I said, I'm not actually sure when the present exists because it is so fleeting!

Perhaps we should just live in history. I suggest we be mindful at all times, for all times, as we create and unfold our own history.

I'm not sure where I got this, or if I made it up:

The Past has no future.
The Future has no past.
The Present has no future nor past.

From a practical standpoint, one day, you are living the perfect life, surfing a great wave, and the next day you experience a seizure and find yourself in the hospital with a diagnosis of stage four lung cancer with metastases to the spine and brain.

One day, you kiss your wife goodbye as she goes to do her community volunteer work; you drop your twelve-year-old boy off at dance class and your ten-year-old daughter at her karate dojo. While on your way to speak at a charity function, you get hit by a drunk driver, and you are killed.

So, I guess even if there doesn't seem to be a measurable "present," it is the best and only place to live—because the moment after "now" can be a life-changer.

Chapter Thirty-Two

Reaper Madness

Death twitches in my ear. "Live," he says, "I am coming."
                                                    —*Virgil*

You've probably heard the old saw "Life is a sexually transmitted disease with a terminal diagnosis."

That fact becomes more and more apparent as we glide through the youthful stages of delusional immortality, past the peaking stages of health, and finally fall into the declining, dysfunctional realm... approaching death.

As we've discussed, all of us have exposure to death in many ways, whether a pet, grandparents, aunts, uncles, parents, friends, reading the news, or simply watching television. Each individual departs at their own time, each in their own way.

Naturally, I was exposed to all of those. But by choosing to become a doctor, I added a whole other collection of witnessed deaths.

From those individuals, I've gathered a few observations that may help you prepare for a great death:

- Start your preparations early by developing a strong spiritual practice and being balanced in body, mind, and spirit. (See the Six Aspects of Optimal Health for guidance.)

- Don't wait until the last minute to take care of your responsibilities.

- Don't leave the responsibility of dealing with your remains to others without talking to them and having instructions in writing. (And on this topic, think of how your remains will affect the environment and plan accordingly.)

- Throughout life, use the metaphor of "the Grim Reaper." As I said, we are all terminal, so the subject of death should not be taboo. Granted, you want the Grim Reaper to remain a shadow or a ghost for as long as possible. The best way to avoid an early meeting is by putting up a protective barrier: the Six Aspects of Optimal Health.

- Write a death poem. Borrowed from the Japanese culture, a death poem (many times in the form of haiku) forces each person to recognize they're going to die. It allows them to reflect on their life and share their feelings about their impending transition.

- Write your eulogy and be sure to add some humor. Add a lot of humor, if you're so inclined.

- If writing a death poem or eulogy is too overwhelming, then at least consider writing your own toe tag (the slip of cardboard they hang on your toe in the morgue).

Just to make everyone laugh and lighten the mood, I recently mulled over the idea of placing something completely absurd on my toe tag: "After my death, refer to me only as 'Cowgirl Jill!' "

I enjoyed imagining the confused looks on everyone's faces and their laughter. Ah, the laughter. I have no doubt some of my friends would comply—to share a final inside joke with me.

Based on a dream I had as a preteen, I believed I would die at an early age—somewhere in my early thirties. I was fine with that. Why? I was so focused on becoming a doctor that it didn't matter to me if I would only be able to practice for a short time. At least I would have been a doctor!

Obviously, my premonition of a short gig was fatally flawed (or rather, not fatal at all). Now, I am a lot older and my terminal status is coming a lot closer. I have done all the things I've recommended to you here, and in some way, I am looking forward to the final curtain. (Or is it final?)

The predominant lesson I learned from a lifetime of witnessing death is to live a great life! Have fun! Do good things! Try not to hurt anyone! Make a difference!

Chapter Thirty-Three

Happy Trails

Be where you are, otherwise,
you will miss your life.

—*Buddha*

I am often asked the question "How should one approach life?"

Think about it: we are not "approaching" life—we are already in it. Instead, the question should be "How should one approach injury, illness, and death?" Because that is where we are headed.

On the path we are born to travel, we know we will live, and we know we will die. No surprises there.

Personally, I look at incense as an analogy for life. As you burn a stick or cone of incense, a metamorphosis occurs at the flame—from concrete to abstract. The solid incense burns; its smoke rises into the clouds and atmosphere; rain forms from those clouds and showers the plants on the earth; the plants grow and are later used to create more incense. Again and again. I believe this is the same metamorphosis we experience in life and death.

However, there are differing opinions of what happens after we die.

Will we be judged on how we lived and be assigned to the appropriate place for eternity? Will we have not learned all our lessons (or not completely eliminated the consequences of our karma) so that we will return again? In either of these cases, it appears that being a good person and learning lessons is of paramount importance.

Some believe we just return to dust. If that is the case, then perhaps it's even more important to adequately utilize this "one time around" to leave a legacy of good.

I'm practical. If indeed we are destined to return to the earth, we are going to be mulch. Endeavor to be the best mulch you can be—eat well.

After the bare requisites of living and reproducing, man wants most to leave some record of himself, a proof, perhaps, that he has really existed.

He leaves his proof on wood, on stone, or on the lives of other people.

This deep desire exists in everyone, from the boy who scribbles on a wall to the Buddha who etches his image in the race mind.

Life is so unreal.

I think that we seriously doubt that we exist and go about trying to prove that we do.

—John Steinbeck

Chapter Thirty-Four

The Final Chapter

 lthough it appears labeled as such—this is not the end of my book.

 Visit **GlennWollman.com/resources** and there you'll find a continuation of my writings—a travelogue of guideposts for your Path of Best Existence.

The sheer act of labeling something doesn't make that label true.

Similarly, how do we know that death is the final chapter in our existence? We don't. And, unfortunately, by the time we do know, we aren't in a position to publish our findings.

Hospice workers, oncologists, nurses, and religious leaders can attest to the privilege of working with the dying. Being in the emergency department allowed me to be a part of the process on so many levels.

I've been in the presence of people of various races, cultures, genders, and ages at the moment of their passing. I have seen people die whimpering and crying, or anxious and in panic.

There were also those who were calm and serene. The ones who were balanced, lived their Missions, worked on self-improvement, and successfully traveled their individual path of best existence usually died with grace.

So, I come full circle and ask the question again: "How should one approach injury, illness, and death?" Everyone gets to make their own choice, but I can bear witness through observation and offer this advice:

Live well; die better.

The key to immortality is first living a life worth remembering.

—*Augustine of Hippo*

Conclusion

Robert Frost took "the road less traveled," and Frank Sinatra did it his way. I have had a great life, creating my "path that didn't exist" and making the right decisions along the way—most of the time.

I sometimes flash back to myself as an excited, inquisitive, yet somewhat helpless third-year medical student, staring at the young boy suffering with a palm frond in his eye. I think of the knowledge and skills I've obtained since then, the experiences, camaraderie, sadness, happiness, and sometimes carnage.

I reflect on all the patients I touched and who touched me. I recall moments in "The Pit" when there were multi-casualty incidents and we were elbows deep in body parts—blood and fluids splattering everywhere.

While others would think my world was extremely stressful, I didn't. At times like those, I stepped back for a moment and thought back to my medical school admission interview. Suddenly, I would realize I was smiling—at my happiest. I loved helping people and working with my hands.

(But by the way, I still can't do anything mechanical.)

I have honored my Gift, recognized and followed my Mission, and remained semi-Responsible in terms of health by honoring the Six Aspects of Optimal Health.

The aspects of Nutrition, Physical Activity, Sleep Management, and Stress Management are perhaps more straightforward. Our Patterns of Behavior are the key to unlocking each aspect, while Spirituality is the connective energy that creates the condition of optimal health for your cells.

I hope I have impressed upon you that cells rule. If you don't treat them well, they know where you live—and they know how to hurt you. In fact, they can kill you. It is when all of your cells die that the you-that-you-think-you-are dies.

Your Gift and your Mission are important, but they need to be protected and nurtured by your Responsibility. If you are in optimal health, honoring your Gift and living your Mission, chances are you will be on your Path of Best Existence.

My closing advice, fellow wayfarers: Take care of your health. Be grateful. Have fun. Do good. Try not to hurt anyone. Make a difference.

Oh, and one final suggestion: While you travel your path in body, mind, and spirit—don't litter!

Epilogue

It was early Monday morning on October 21, 2019. I was busily putting the final editing tweaks on a few items Glenn and I had discussed by email the night before. We were due to have our weekly phone meeting in a few hours.

That's when I got the call from his wife, and my friend, Heidi.

Glenn had passed away overnight.

As Glenn's editor, I collaborated with him via the internet on a shared document of this manuscript. As each of us would make changes, the other could accept or reject the changes. Glenn loved to joke that I enjoyed rejecting him. Sometimes, he would think of absurd things to add... just to wait for my rejection.

It became our game.

Believe me, my outright rejections were few and far between; I hung on his every word. More often than not, the seeming rejection was a software glitch—a mistaken notation that a "cut-and-paste" of his priceless information was gone. Glenn knew that, but nonetheless, he continued to tease me.

As I spoke to his wife on the phone, I silently told Glenn, "I reject this! You can't be gone! Rejection! REJECTION!!"

Looking back on our time working together, I feel incredibly privileged to have learned from Glenn. His guidance helped me on my own path, medically, spiritually, and philosophically. His viewpoint on life was astounding. He saw the beauty in everything, every moment, everyone. He equally appreciated both knowledge and mystery. He was a true Renaissance man who cared deeply about all life—big and small.

I am happy we were able to complete the work on his book before he passed. With the exception of a few minor additions of transcribed telephone conversations, this is the book as Glenn saw it. This is his vision. His legacy.

Oddly, the section that had given us the most difficulty was Part Four—the chapters on death. It dawned on me as I tried to make sense of the news: Leave it to Glenn. He went to do the research.

I have no doubt he will try to send me the answers.

Or maybe I'll be visited by an inexplicable crow to whom I'll say:

"Until we meet again, 'Cowgirl Jill,' be the best mulch you can be. Thank you for allowing me to inhabit your mind, if only a very small part of it for a very brief time. I will remain forever blessed. I love you."

—Tracey Davis

Acknowledgments

This book was assembled by sewing together decades of Glenn's scribbles, organizing his memories, thoughts and knowledge. Tracey, you are the brave soul who not only took on this journey, but spent years of your life inside of his head. You may have gotten a glimpse of his appreciation for you; that was but the tip of the iceberg. The joy you gave him over the years you worked together was immeasurably massive. I cannot thank you enough. Your only face-to-face meeting with Glenn was so random and so improbable that I believe your connection was (and is) something otherworldly.

Glenn would fill these pages with the names of all the nurses, caregivers, educators and healers who he worked with, learned from, and was treated by. If you knew Glenn, you know it's what he'd do. The most I can do is bow to you in gratitude.

I personally would like to acknowledge Kathleen and Segovia. You both went above and beyond anyone in your fields of expertise. You patiently dealt with my ignorance of anything books, along with my tears and fears every step of this journey. Your empathy blows my mind and fills me with gratitude.

Carol, Penny, Dennis, Emily, Don and Vahan. You kept me sane. No small feat.

With undying love and appreciation,
Heidi